# The Dandy Dieter



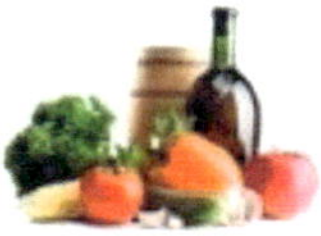

## Thick or Thin?

Judith Jacobs Schwartz

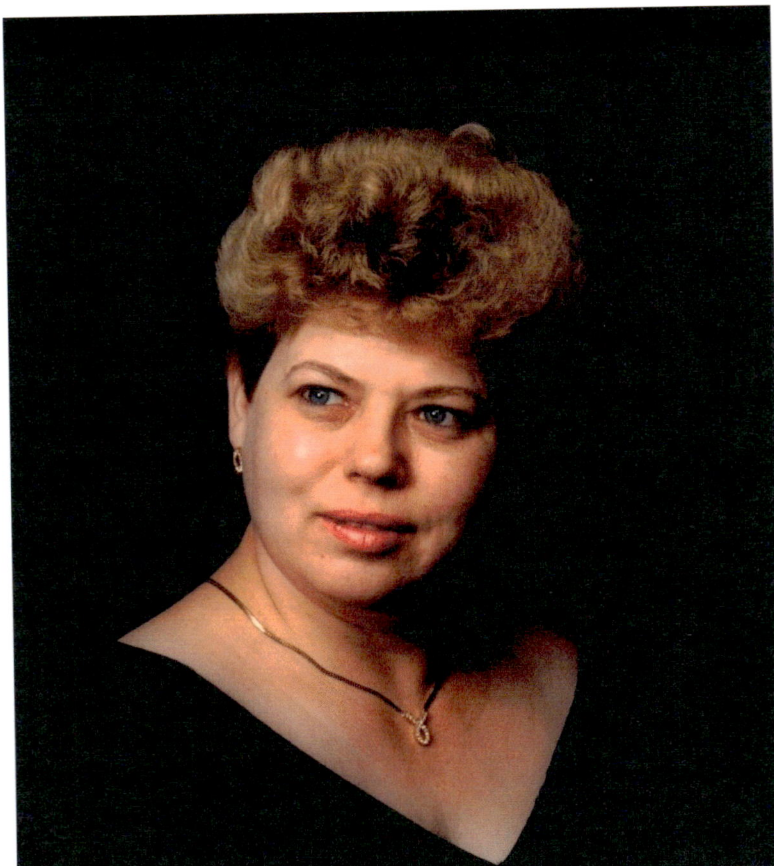

Judith Ann Jacobs Schwartz

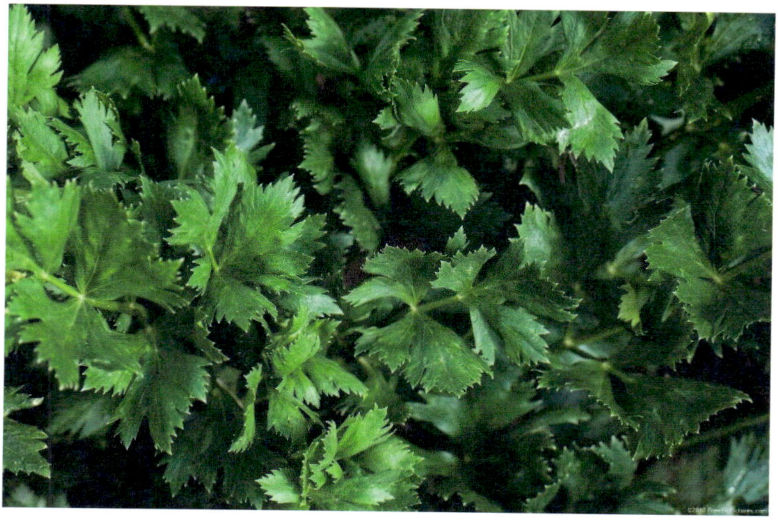

# The Dandy Dieter

**Written and illustrated in parts by Author**
**Judith Jacobs Schwartz**
**JudySchwartzGifts.Com**

Printed in the United States of America
Angelee Coleman Grider, Editor
M.O.R.E. Publishers CO - Memphis (TN)
ISBN 978-0-692-27449-1 Library of Congress Control Number: 2014916267

| | | |
|---|---|---|
| D | **Dear Lord, help me.** | 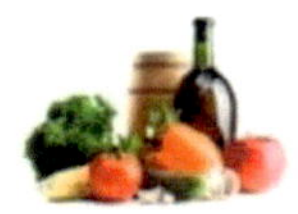 |
| I | **I can do this:** | |
| E | **eat smaller portions,** | |
| T | **think thin,** | |
| E | **exercise,** | |
| R | **remember to thank God for all of His help.** | |
| S | **Special am I, in a smaller size.** | |

*Dear Readers,*

*If you have ever been on a diet, you will want to read this book.*

*The word "diet" can make you hurt somebody. Then one cookie can calm you down, and put your nerves at ease.*

*This book will give you a laugh, or two and some snack tips to keep you from being hungry all of the time. You will feel like a million dollars when you start losing weight.*

*You will see recipes that you can share with your friends. Make bets to see who can lose the most weight.*

*We know that being heavy is not fun, but who said that you can't laugh while you are losing the weight. Remember, you don't have to diet until you die. Try going on a diet and you just might "die" when you see yourself in the mirror three sizes smaller.*

*In this book, carrots will guide you to the finish line. Good luck on your diet. Your diet is now in God's hands.*

*Judith Jacobs Schwartz*
*St. Louis, MO*

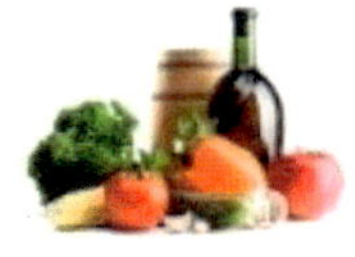

## Contents





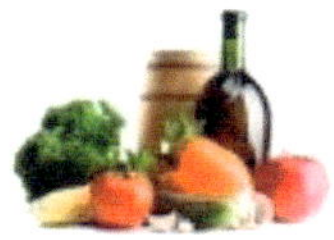

# *The Dandy Dieter*

*If you can grab a slab,*
*quick, text God…*
*{but not while you are driving}*

*Judith Jacobs Schwartz*

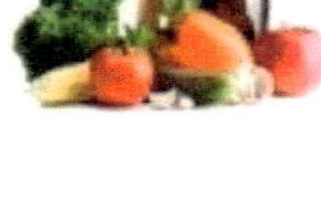

# *I Dedicate This Book*

## *To my dear mother*

## *and*

*To all those who found out what a jelly donut tastes like; what the crunch of potato chips sounds like; and what a hot slice of pizza feels like going down your throat.*

*Can you smell the fresh baked bread?*

*This book is to help you put the butter on "it" and then throw "it" into the trash can.*

*If you can do that,*
*you just might be saved.*

*I would like to dedicate this book to all those who, when they sit on a chair, their "cornbread" hangs over the sides.*

*I did not write this book to offend anyone, but to give all the dieters a laugh and to get a fresh start for a body of which to be proud.*

*Good luck and may God knock the steak-burger*
*right out of your hand.*

# The Dieter's Prayer

The dieter's prayer was written with humor, and to encourage anyone who is trying to lose weight.

"THE PRAYER"
Oh Lord, please bless my fat.
I know just right where it's at.
I love my cookies and donuts,
but I eat them with celery and carrots.
I promise that I won't cry
when I can't eat fries.
Lord, please help me to put on my seat belt
and get back on the right road.
Lord calm down the hunger in my stomach.
Give me the power to pass up the junk food,
and to kick my pizza to the curb.
Help me to put my candy in the trash,
to lose this weight, and to make it last.
With your help Lord,
I can do this.
A new size is on the way.
My goal weight is
whatever I want it to be.
Please Lord, don't leave me now.
My fat is in your hands.

God bless.

Enjoy my book.

Chapter 1

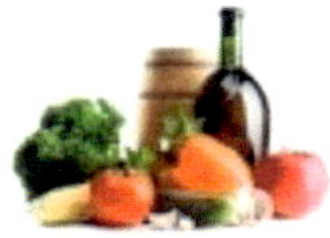

# The Dandy Dieter

Okay high thighs, here we go again to start another diet. I'll be right back. I have to go in the other room to laugh my head off (sniff, sniff).

Okay, I'm back. So how many diets have you tried? How old did you say you are? You think the word "diet" is your middle name? You feel that you have been on a diet forever?

We know what the right foods are and we eat them. Yet do we eat them with donuts, cookies, crackers and peanut butter, potato chips...? Got the picture?

Okay, you starving people who look as if you are the refrigerator and everything in it, let's get started. Now how much weight do you want to lose? Well, if you have been big for the past ten years, you should lose enough weight so that your pants slip off your hips, and hit the floor. Now does that sound like enough weight? Sounds good to me.

Did you have a talk with the diet devil and tell him that he is not going to win this time, and to back off? First, go shopping and load up on all of the greens that the shopping cart can hold. Then go over to the fruit section and pick some apples and oranges. Can you get the rest without me? Good. Now we mean tough business.

Back off thin people. Here I come. I'm on my way to the body shop. It would be nice if we could go to the body shop and order a new set of hips and new buttocks. That way this diet would be on hold.

Time to jump on the scale and see how bad the old "bod" is. Now do you still want to knock off a pizza? How many of you have high blood pressure or high blood sugar? If you lose about twenty pounds, your blood pressure and your high blood sugar would go down. When you gain, the pressure and the sugar level go up. Then you will have other problems. Wouldn't you like to feel and look better? Now is the best time. Think about it for a while.

I am so tired of being hungry. I can see a cheeseburger on television and gain eight pounds just by sitting in the chair. I gain three pounds if I see a candy wrapper on the ground. God, I need a cookie fast.

We seem to always have food on the brain. You need a nice hobby to keep you busy. Go to the gym. Meet new people. Plant some flowers in the backyard. Hang around with people bigger than you are, and you will be the thin one.

Giving up the good stuff is not easy. Trying to eat a sandwich without bread is not so great. Whenever I see a thin person eat like a horse, I wonder what it would be like to be able to eat anything and be thin. Is that a blessing or what? Well, back to the celery and carrots.

Some people say "Eat lots of fruits and vegetables". So who wants to turn green for Christmas? Fruit is good for us, but pizza tastes better. We need will-power against the cookies and donuts. I bet you can do this if you really want to do so. Go on and surprise your friends and see their lips drop when they see that you have lost some weight. Watch for the diet devil. He is after you. Put that hot dog in the trash and don't forget the bun. Remember that a thinner derriere can walk faster. So don't run to the kitchen and eat everything on which you can get your hands.

It's break time. So go to the bathroom and meet me back here on this page in five minutes. I must get me a peach.

I'm waiting. Where are you? I hope that you didn't stuff down about nine cookies and a glass of milk.

Now what do you think is harder than being on a diet? I know. The answer is "paying taxes and staying married longer than ten years". Maybe this is not so hard after all. It could be worse. I just know that there is a trick to this madness. I know a girl who was on a diet for so long until she began to act a little crazy. I guess she was eating all of the wrong foods. A diet can make you go nuts if you let it. The world has its portion of nuts already.

So say a prayer, and get back on track. God, please help me to control myself at the salad bar. Wouldn't you like to go to the salad bar and put real food on your plate besides lettuce and cottage cheese? Why do we have salad bars anyway? It's probably just to keep the diet devil busy.

Did you ever wonder what it would be like if you could eat anything you wanted, and never have to worry about gaining weight? To me that would be a life-time blessing.

I just love sweets, chips, and all of the stuff that help one put on the extra pounds. For example, if you lose about eight pounds, then you gain back four. Don't be sad and let that disappointment discourage you. I know that there is a long line of dieters fighting. Maybe we weigh ourselves too much. How about just weighing once a week? Give your body a chance to get use to the new eating pattern and then maybe the pounds will come off a little faster. Don't forget to do some bends and stretches now and then. Every little bit helps.

Some dieters say to drink a lot of water. I drank so much water until I thought that I was going to drown. I can't even swim. I lost two days of my life because I was in the bathroom reading. When I came out, I think the water-drinking had to take a rest.

Watch the labels on fruit juice. It is full of sugar. Don't fill up on crackers. They will blow you up when you drink a glass of water. I know. Now let's read the rest of the "no, no list":

sweets,
chips,
no pasta,
red meat only once a week,
no bread, and
no crying on the bread.

The "no, no lists is full of goodies. When you really look at it, the list has all of the stuff we are eating right? Okay, are you getting hungry just reading this book?

Well, don't feel too bad because your day is not too far away. Your mirror sadness will turn into a mirror of victory with a big smile, hold on and hang in there. There is a lot of work to do.

You may think, "I just can't do this diet another day". Well baby, you can do it. Now close your eyes. Do you see yourself in a pretty blue dress? Your outfit has white sandals and a tiny little waist. Okay, that feels good doesn't it? Now there is the picture of a beautiful lady. Now open up your eyes. The diets are on once again.

Notice that your doctor will always tell you to lose weight. Do doctors think for one minute that if we knew how to lose the weight, we would not go to see the Doctor with the LARGE body?

So God, help us and bless us along the way. Keep your seat belts on because it is a long road. Let's tell the diet devil to go down another road. Leave us alone! We are on a mission!

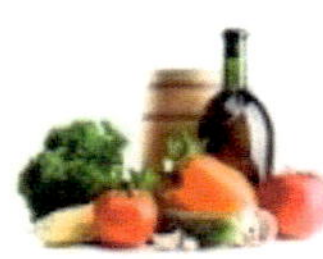

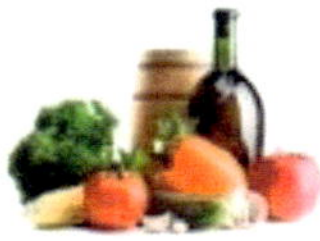

Chapter 2

# Know When To Diet

1. When you are going somewhere and your belly gets there before you do
2. When you are taking a shower, you drop the soap, or you bend down to pick it up, and say "Excuse me."
3. When you are walking down the street and it starts to get dark – You feel that someone is following you, so you walk a little faster. Then you stop and turn around to realize that it's just the shadow of your "big behind".
4. When you are sitting in a chair; you feel that somebody is sitting on your lap, but you look down and nobody is there
5. When you see yourself without clothes and you reach for a pain pill
6. When you start walking like a duck
7. When you sit on a chair; your feet go to sleep before you do
8. When you start to take a bubble bath; you sit into the tub and there are no bubbles
9. When you bend over to pick up something, and rip the seams in your pants
10. When you stand up and your belly hangs to one side

It's time to find a diet and get going! Let's face it. We are not built like Barbie Dolls, and if God wanted all of us to be thin, He wouldn't have given us the good stuff. Let's burn the brownies and pass up the chocolate cake.

Say constantly, "May God bless my body and help me to reach my goal."

## Know Why You Should Diet

1. To feel better
2. To look better
3. So you can touch your toes
4. To have better health
5. To live longer
6. To fit into the outfit hanging in your closet for the past ten years
7. So you can wear nice outfits that are on sale
8. So you can walk with your head up high instead of your thighs
9. Because you step on scales, hear a bell and you know it's not the doorbell
10. So you can shock your whole dysfunctional family (I'm sure everybody has one person in their family, who at times you thought was just not right – no names please)
11. Because you are worth the effort to be your best
12. So you will be able to walk a while and not run out of breath
13. So you won't take up two seats on the airplane
14. So when you get into bed the mattress will not yell "help!"
15. So that after you take a shower, you won't need two towels for drying

If you can think of any other reasons, pass them on to others.

We know all of the food that we can't eat because that is our everyday diet. Right? We can do this once and for all, or we will have to rent a U-

Haul. Now that really got my attention. How about you? Did you pass out thinking about riding in the back of the U-Haul? Don't make a doctor's appointment yet. You can still be saved.

Okay chicken liver, let's go. Then get the trash can and follow me. We don't need these potato chips nor these two boxes of cookies... What about this peanut butter jar? Now that the trash can is full of all the "good stuff," let's talk about the stuff that we can eat.

We can eat lots of fruit, but watch all of the sugar in the canned fruit. Pears are good. I like apples and oranges. How about you? How are we doing so far? You can eat an orange while you are reading and you won't feel so bad. Let's eat grapes for a snack. We can have wheat crackers and a slice of cheese. How about sliced cucumbers, a glass of skimmed milk, and one cookie of your choice? I said one cookie. Drop the other four.

For breakfast, we can have one-half of an English muffin with sugar-free jam, and a half cup of coffee with no sugar and just a little cream. This will fill you up, and then you can eat a small snack in about four hours.

For snack, we can have a few Graham Crackers and a glass of skim milk. Okay, time out. Let's be back here in five minutes.

I'm back. Are you there? How did you do on your break? Did you down a sandwich and drink a soda? If so, shame on you. Now think of all the reasons why you want to be thinner. If you eat smaller portions and drink water, you will be surprised at how fast you will fill up your stomach. I think that the hardest thing is to go to a holiday party and not be able to eat the good stuff than can make you hurt someone, and they wouldn't even know why.

Caution. A person on a diet can get mean. They say things that they don't mean. They can hurt your feelings. They are not bad people, it's like taking a bone away from a Great Dane. Don't think he won't tear you up quickly.

The situation is also like when you can't eat cookies. It can destroy the whole day, and nobody will not even know you are on a diet but you and God. Please eat the darn cookie, and deal with it. Okay, do we feel a little better? I am so glad.

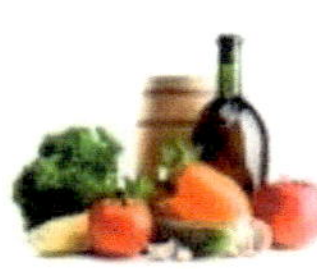

Chapter 3

# What To Eat?

Look at that "thin list". It includes carrots, celery, peppers, and lettuce. So get your spoon and dig in, but don't forget the dressing. Truthfully, I am so tired of carrots. I think that I have hair growing between my toes. Yet, how about baked chicken with a baked potato? Sounds good? You can eat turkey, tuna – oh Lord the tuna. I eat so much tuna until I feel like a fish. Now I don't like to go fishing.

You can eat Graham Crackers with skim milk. Now that makes me want to run to the table. So what is your favorite food? How do you feel about giving it up? You can always have dry cereal and ice water.

Okay, now let's get down to business. Salad is good. How about tomatoes and onions? You can eat some of the good stuff, but it's how much you eat.

Get a smaller plate, no seconds, and eat small so you can stop when you are full. Don't stuff yourself just because food is left on your plate.

Calories add up fast, so watch the small things such as cookies, crackers, nuts and popcorn. Watch the carbs too. They turn into sugar and that can mean trouble with your blood. I use to have high-blood pressure. I took a pill every morning.

Then I said to myself, "If it bothers me, I can get rid of it." After a while, I did not have high blood pressure. But this may not work for everyone. So don't get rid of your husband just yet. You may need him to open a jar.

Can you think of good snacks to fill you up? I eat wheat crackers, diet with a friend, and make a bet. See who can lose the most weight in four months, then go for another four months. Don't make yourself sick, but eat proteins and fiber. Watch the bread. Get use to drinking cold water, not sodas. This will help a lot. Good luck and say a prayer. God is watching.

Now, I know that it is not easy to be on a diet. If you have ever been on a diet, you know what I mean.

Let's share some more of the foods that we can eat to help us. We can eat raisins. Munch on a cup of pears. An apple will fill you up and burn the fat faster than anything that I know. Apples taste good. Munch on Trail Mix with nuts, fruit, cereal, with maybe pretzels. They are good. Eat a piece of chicken with a salad and a bowl of Jell-O. I like orange juice with orange slices included. You can cut up fresh strawberries and put them in Jell-O. Now that is real good. You can have a small turkey sandwich with a tomato and a few wheat crackers with a small salad. Do you know that if you eat the right food, your body will get use to it and in time, you won't even miss the food that you ate before the diet? You have to eat the same food for the rest of your life and you will have a better chance the fat won't come back.

Now, here is a way to save calories. When you eat out, order a large glass of ice water and ask for a slice of lemon. You are probably thinking, "What about the soda?" Well, it's not on your list for one thing. You have to eat differently so get use to it if you want to be thin.

As I said before, dieting is not easy. If it was easy, everybody would be thin and nobody would ever have to be on a diet. That felt good just trying that line. But we are not going to get off that easy. How many are still with me? I know that I lost a few readers who gave up for a large bowl of ice cream. We will see you for the holidays. You can't get thin with prayer alone. You have to sweat and give up the high-calorie foods.

Is there a family member who is on the heavy side? Do you see the pain they are in trying to lose weight? Food is also an illness for some people. They just can't stop eating no matter what they do. Before they know it, they are three hundred pounds. It seems that they got large in no time. There was too much food, and no hobby; maybe, too much idle time and they have no outside interests. You can't do this alone. There is help waiting. Keep them in your prayers, and ask God to help them to lose weight and to be healthy.

How about the good stuff like chips and dip, cheese and crackers? Sink your teeth into a BLT (bacon/bologna, lettuce and tomato) sandwich. Have you had enough yet? Well this is what makes your body spread out and never come back to its real shape. My, did that stuff taste good? So how did we get fat in the first place?

We used our mouth. We stuff everything in it, all morning long, and then all of a sudden it's lunch time. Do you really feel hungry? Or are you just eating because everybody else is eating? So say a prayer and God will help you pitch the chips and dip in the ditch. Look at the calories you will save. The only one that is getting fatter is the bag lady. Now fight temptation. So put on your right blinker, buzz up to the drive-up, and order the biggest cheeseburger and fries. The devil is laughing at you. Don't let him get away with that. When you go around the corner, toss the good stuff out of the window in the ditch. Get a grip on yourself, and drive away with a smile on your face. I am so proud of you. Let some thin person tell you how good the fries were. Nobody goes to the ditch to check out the good stuff but the bag lady.

You will have days that you just can't take it anymore. You lose control over a simple thing as a slice of hot pizza. Okay, don't spit on yourself. We know what it tastes like. We just have to take a breath and think of the reasons why we want to be thin. Then start a better day and eat right. Be glad we have God on our side. We can only do this for ourselves. Nobody else can do it for us. I always wondered that when we try so hard why we can't go the rest of our lives without the "good stuff".

Do we just beat up ourselves forever, or what? This is not easy, and don't listen to the guy that says it is. They look like they never been on a diet in their whole life. That's why their finger nails look so darn good. Be proud and try. Get up in the morning and say a prayer for that day, and every day. If you need some help, go in the bathroom and look in the mirror and say "This is my year to be thin." Don't get crazy and eat the whole tube of toothpaste either. If you don't lose any weight, at least your teeth will sparkle.

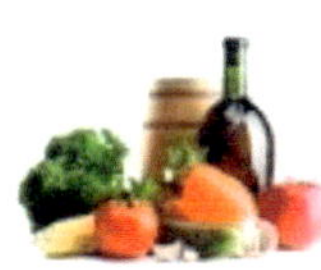

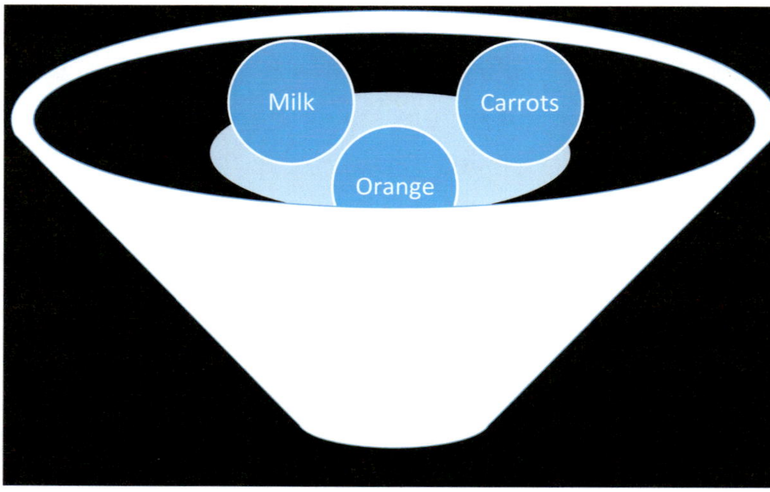
Milk
Carrots
Orange

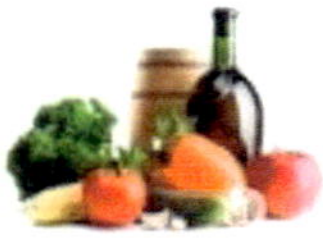

Chapter 4

# The Body of Exercise

Are you tired of people telling you to exercise? Well, me too. My body is so beat up that when I exercise, I end up in the doctor's office. How about you? I tried to exercise my legs and I couldn't walk for about two days. I'm sure that you have also been there.

Jump rope. It will shake up your brain so you won't know if you are hungry or not. When is the last time you did any exercise at all? What did you say? 1990? What? You better get off that couch and bend a little. If your lips turn purple, sit back down and take four deep breaths.

Well, did we learn anything new other than that a diet stinks? We can pray a lot, eat celery a lot, and we can really try to fool the family. I would just like to see the faces on my sisters. I have two and they are both thin, but I was blessed with the best legs. At least God helped me with something. I'm sure everybody has one good body part. What is yours? God didn't forget to give us special blessings. We just have to find them.

When you lose your first ten pounds, you can go and buy yourself something new. Then for the next ten pounds, you can have a special dinner out on the town. By then, you will know how to order. You are on your way, so dress up for the ride.

Now is the time to clean out all of the heavy clothes in the closet. However, save some of the clothes in case we put back on a few pounds. We will have those days, but keep on eating the right stuff. You will be able to move a little faster with less weight.

Now lie on the floor, and swing your right leg up. Touch your toes. Take it slowly or your face will stay that color purple. I like purple, but what I would like more is to breathe better. Do this now and then and when you get up, I hope that the fat stays on the floor. May carrots and celery travel. Definitely send chips and burgers in the ditch.

I know that you really want to lose about thirty pounds, and you just can't get the fat off. Well, the world is full of people just like you. Don't forget me. I'm in line too. I do like carrots, but I can't eat them for the rest of my life. My face will turn orange.

I see these people running down the sidewalk with their ear phones, and sweat is all over their body, not to mention that it's about 102 outside. I wonder what keeps them from falling in a ditch. I just imagine that the next day when I'm watching the news, the broadcaster will be telling about the body that was found in the ditch. I will say, "Oh, my God. I saw him running yesterday. You have to be careful or you can hurt yourself."

"Why can't somebody invent a safe way to burn off this fat?" Think about it. They can put a man on the moon, but they can't help us with the weight problems. I wonder if there are fat people in heaven. Every day is a new day. Some are good and some are really bad. Yet you feel like you did pretty good one day, but watch out for the next day.

We just have to toss the candy bars in the ditch, or don't buy them at all. Just munch on another carrot. May God bless our bodies. So keep up the good work. Thin is on the way!

Do you ever go to a party and all the food is on the "NO, NO LIST"? So what do you eat – one chip, one piece of cheese, one piece of meat, and a small glass of water? Then you can party until your behind falls off. Later, go home and make like you never went. Even when you lose some weight, you will never be able to eat like that again. Your whole eating will be different. Find new things to eat that will make you feel full as if you are not on a diet.

How about cereal with peaches? Do you like fish? I do like tuna, but not all of the time. Salads – I do like and salads are good for you.

Look in other people shopping carts to see what they are buying. Look in cookbooks, and get some new ideas of good dishes to eat. Don't forget the carrots. They are back-up for hungry pains. Do you like grapes? They are good for you. I like them in cereal. Ask other dieters what they eat and maybe you will like the same things. Whatever you eat, just eat half and you will fill up faster. In time, you will have half of a body. If you see a real hunk walking down the street, you will have a great bod' to turn his head. I bet that's been a while, right?

Come on, we know that it's hard to lose weight. You can eat dirt, sugar-free of course, but if you don't do some exercise, nothing will happen. I guess you know that by now. You cannot fool fat. It won't burn if you don't light the fire. Your body has to sweat all of the meanness out of you, so you can focus on the calories that you can't eat. That even made me hungry. Oh well, back to a day with no donuts.

I have my days when I feel like eating nothing. I think, "Why bother?" You can only eat so many carrots, right?

I couldn't sleep the other night. I tossed and turned all night. I closed my eyes and there I was - like a real nut counting carrots. I would have counted eighty-seven but I think I ate two of them in my sleep. I think you can gain weight in your sleep by dreaming about the bake sale. I can almost taste the jelly rolls. God woke me up just so I wouldn't eat the darn things.

I had a dream that I was locked inside of a chocolate factory. You know the rest. I ate so much chocolate until my family didn't know who I was at the Christmas party. For once I knew what it felt like being an outsider. At the Christmas party I brought some carrots just for back up. I sat as far away from the dessert table as possible. Nobody knew who I was sitting so close to the coats.

Get ready for the holidays in a smaller size, and the whole family will want your picture. You will want one too just in case it all comes back. Have a real nice holiday and don't forget to eat like a very small child.

You have worked hard on this diet, so now you can have a piece of cake. How is it going so far? It should taste like heaven in cupcake land. I know that you enjoyed that. So back to the carrots.

There are heavy people who dress so good. They carry their large size very well. Some people carry it well, and some don't. In what group are you? Now it's time for a break. You go to the bathroom and I have to get another beer. I will meet you back here in five minutes.

Okay, I'm back. Where are you? Get out of that kitchen and drop that ham sandwich on the floor. Spit that cookie out of your mouth. We are going to talk about all of the foods that you are trying to eat.

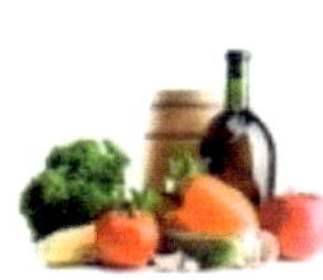

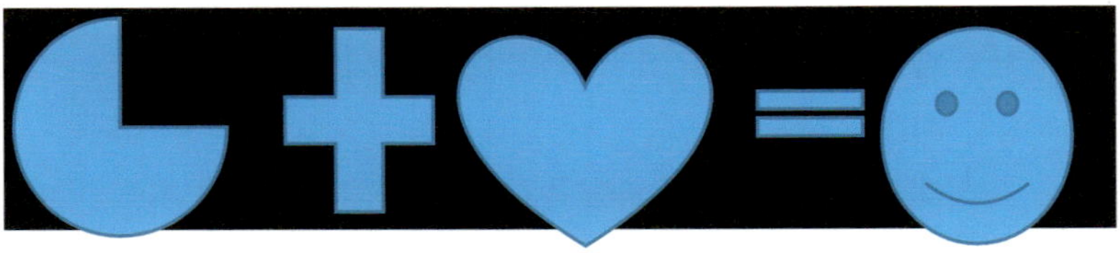

Eating lightly plus a willing heart, equals a satisfied dieter.

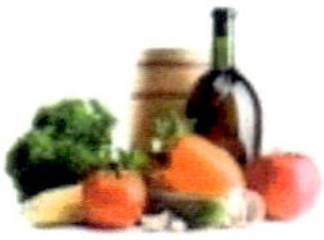

Chapter 5

# Food Or Fat

So you are thinking, "What is food?" and "What is fat?" Well it's simple. You eat food and then you get fat. However, if you eat less food, you get thin. That sounds better already, doesn't it?

Well, take a deep breath and take a bite of salad. Now did that taste good? You can do this. I will push you along and by the end of this year, you will be thinner. Okay? It's time to eat.

Try some figs, yogurt, plain popcorn, baked turkey, cantaloupe, brown rice, salad, cucumbers, applesauce and anything else that you like within reasonable calories. Keep in mind that these will burn off fat. If you get hungry at night, pick things such as peaches, apples, nuts, bell peppers, Graham Crackers, and skim milk. These will fill you up. Try these sometimes.

I know you want to be thin. Can you see the look on your friends' faces when they see you about thirty pounds lighter. Oh how proud you will be. So, if you help me, I will help you, but you first.

You have to keep busy. Clean the bathroom. Get the wash caught up, or do some crafts. Plant some flowers in the back yard. What do you really like to do? Don't make eating food your top activity. It's not.

Get your mind on a hobby and see how many things you can do. You can make money making things with your own ideas, if you keep busy. It will be better to deal with the diet. When you have to stop and get something to eat because you are so hungry from being busy doing a project, that's better than thinking of food all day, and what you can eat next.

Food, or Fat? See the difference? I have been on diets and lost weight, but I am just like you. I can go so long and the good stuff gets the best of me.

Have you seen someone in your family who has lost about thirty-five pounds, and then four months down the line, you see them and they have gained the weight all back? It's hard enough to lose weight. Now we have to find out how to keep the weight off. If you know, e-mail me right away at fastfoods@calories.com

Are you getting hungry, and don't know what to eat? I have been there too, and I always eat things such as grapes, or a slice of rye bread with cheese on it. Does that sound very good? It's not too bad. Did you ever use lettuce for bread? Wrap some tuna with onions in the lettuce and put a slice of tomato on it with a little bit of cheese. Now that really tastes good. Try it! When you go out to eat, you can always pick out the dieters. They are smiling while eating a nice salad. Then their faces turn a pretty purple as they stare at the steak and potatoes on the next table.

There has got to be a pill for this. I hope that I don't die before they get the pill on the market. Just think. You can take a little pill and your belly goes almost flat. Before you know it, you are in a size twelve. That sounds good to me. How about you?

We know that the little pill is never going to be, so back to the carrots and celery. Did you ever wonder what you look like in a size twelve? Nobody could get that smile off your face. You would have more room behind the wheel while driving. You could dress a whole lot better and be so proud of yourself. This all sounds good but this is not an easy thing to do. Right?

I know you have a sad look on your face, but let's face it, if you eat like you want to eat, you will get bigger. We just want to know the trick to this madness. Is there even a trick at all?

To be on a diet, you must count calories, watch the carbs, eat no sugar, nor bread, nor lunchmeat on buns, nor sweets. Now that could make you kill somebody. You better be at least ten feet away from a dieter, or you won't be home for the holidays. Diets do things to people. Take a cookie away from a dieter, and run for your life! I like the dieter who says, "I haven't eaten any food all day." You think, "They must have eaten the kid next door. Well something was creeping down their throat. I guess that is the secret."

What would you do if the doctor tells you to lose some weight, right? Why do you think that he backs up every time you lose another eight pounds when he has to check you for your next appointment? I say that every eight pounds that you lose, makes you a little more dangerous. You are now healthier! Soon the doctor's bill will dwindle. Start smiling. You know the dieters by sight – they are the ones with big smiles while they are gritting their teeth. So back off and beware. Throw them a cookie and run.

First, let's talk about your problem. Do you start off good and then say, "Well maybe one cookie won't hurt?"

Can you eat one cookie, but not the second, third, or the fourth one? Now that's real power. Can I buy some? You can eat two figs and then drink a little water. By the way, watch the ice cream. I know that it's hard to deal with ice cream. However, ice cream will spread your behind way out real fast.

You can fill up by drinking skim milk, and then you can munch on cherries, mangos, nuts and blueberries. But are you thinking, “I do eat all of that stuff, and I am always hungry.”

Maybe you are not eating proteins. I hope you can find something that will fill you up and make you feel better. Nobody wants to feel hungry all of the time. This is your turn to be thin. I have the candles burning. At least something is burning. We need more pretty ladies in this world, so get going baby. If you see me on the street, and you have lost weight, just smile because I will be so proud for you. I’m sure the road was rough.

You have to sweat, do some exercises, give up the good stuff, find a new way to eat for the rest of your life and ask God to help you all of the way through. You can still eat a cookie once in a while, and have a slice of bread now and then. It’s the large hamburgers and fries, the pasta, and the pizza that need to go.

I think I’m on the NO – NO list. I was getting hungry just typing the words. Well how are you doing with all of the diet advice? I don’t know all of the answers, but I do know about the battle of the bulge.

I have seen so many people struggle to lose weight. So what? They lost thirty or forty pounds. They look so good and different. But the next time you see them, they will have gained it all back.

Have you been down that road? We need a different path to take, right? I do know that it’s harder to lose when you get older. I start to tell people that God put too much clay on me when he made me, and that's why some skinny person is walking around with no behind. I guess it's just as hard for thin people to gain a few pounds, as it is for us to lose. Maybe we can sell them a truck load. Let them eat carrots and celery for a while and see how they like it.

Remember to bend, bend, bend! You will be thin, thin, thin.

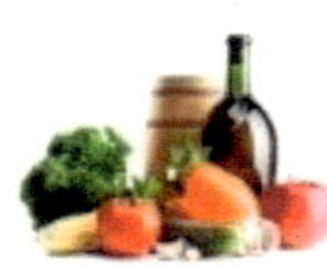

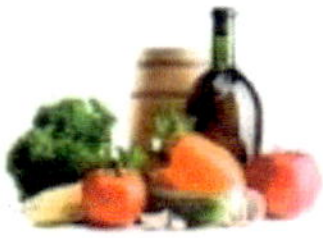

Chapter 6

# A Diet Is Not Fun

Come on, nobody likes to be on a darn diet. We would like to eat anything we want. We would also like to walk down the street with a slim body and turn as many heads as we can.

Do you think that God is testing us with this extra-large body? Well maybe so, but don't count on it. God didn't make us fat. He just gave us the good food that taste so good. We have to be strong and have a little will-power.

***Be Ye Thankful!*** Did you ever try to help a friend to lose some weight, but couldn't do it yourself? Do I have any hands up? I thought so.

Well, some people can stop eating bread for three weeks and drop ten pounds. I'm not one of those people. How about you? Can you drop ten pounds in a short time? If so, please e-mail me and tell me what you are eating.

Also, do you get tired of being the biggest person at the party? Then you watch all of the girls dance and swing their hips when you haven't seen your hips in twelve years, or longer. You know that you do have hips. You just can't find them.

Now, do we need a reason to be on a diet? If you have to sit down to see your toes, there is something going on with your body. When you stand up, do your toes disappear? Do you need another reason to be on a diet? Okay, try this. Have you ever gone into the dressing room to try something on and thought something was wrong with the mirror? You are too thin. Then you think, "I don't remember picking up a Barbie Doll blouse." But the thin YOU feels so good.

Diet days are waiting for your body. So get going and diet until your clothes fall off. Make a doctor's appointment first. Tell him to put on the coffee because you will be bringing the "rolls".

When you go shopping, do you ever see a well-dressed lady who really stands out? You could be that lady, if you wanted to do so. I know that saying it and doing it are not the same. Losing weight is the furry for many people who have to deal with a weight-problem. Some just get so sick of being heavy.

Do you remember when you were thinner? What was going on in your life that kept your mind off food? Do you think about food before you go to bed? Is food on your mind when you wake up in the morning? Now that is a real problem.

Things of interest can keep your mind off of food. Take a short walk. Paint something. Keep yourself busy, and don't be idle. Did you ever think of going to Heaven and God says to you, "My child, what did you do on earth? Tell me about your accomplishments." Then you stand there in complete silence.

A busy person will have a lot to say. I am one of them. They will have to get a court-order to shut my mouth because I'm always busy. Never-the-less, the time here on earth is so special and so short. You want to get the most out of it.

Happiness is not bought in a box. You have to make it happen, and it comes with hard work. You have to suffer to get what you want in life, and that is not easy. We can pray, but we have to work at it, and not give up.

I have lost the same weight over and over and I do know the pain that comes with being heavy. I get so tired of the "NO, NO List," and not being able to eat the good stuff. I'm sure you are tired too.

However, we can start another day, and this time break the mirror. If you eat small, then go and find something to do. Don't sit for hours. Think of ways to keep busy. So what do you say? Is this your year to be thin, and show off your new you?

Put down that pizza, and pick up that carrot. The food problem is going to get shaken up. I hope that you will really try this time and don't forget that you will have better health. God is on your side. He won't forget when you are eating your carrots. It just takes time.

Good luck and fill up the ditch with all of the good stuff. Think of it this way, if you can lose about thirty pounds before Christmas, I bet Santa would like for you to sit on his lap, and you wouldn't even break his knees. Go Girl!

Now is the time to count all of our blessings. I don't mean that burger and the onion rings you just stuffed in your mouth. Anything that tastes that good goes in the trash can. We know that it is hard to throw the good stuff in the trash can. I bet you can't guess who is willing to take out the trash? Do we have an idea of what we are going to eat for breakfast?

Let's make this easy on our nervous system. Now remember this is going to be foods we can eat for the rest of our lives. If you don't like oatmeal, don't sit at the table and gag. Change it to something you like. Forced-eating is one of the main problems. In other words, you eat eggs, or oatmeal to lose weight but you really don't like them. Right?

Put something on your plate that you do like. You can eat that for the rest of your life, but don't waste your day with something you don't even like.

Try a few weeks of eating things you don't like and somebody could get hurt. I hope that it's not me. I see that you are going to eat one-half of a grapefruit, a small English muffin with sugar-free jam on it, a small tomato, and a half cup of coffee with a little skim milk. This you can live with, and not beat up your nerves.

In four hours, you should eat a snack. How about a small apple with a few Graham Crackers, and a glass of skim milk? Okay, so far, how do you feel? Is it time for lunch already?

Let's have a half cup of tuna in a leaf of lettuce, a small salad with tomatoes, and a small orange with a glass of skim milk.

Now for the last meal of the day, try a small baked chicken breast, a small portion of mashed potatoes, a half cup of corn and a cup of peaches. You can also try coffee, tea or skim milk of your choice.

At seven o'clock tonight, nibble on a few wheat crackers with a slice of cheese, and a glass of iced tea. Eat nothing after seven o'clock. Drink only liquids such as tea or water. After you change the foods around for each meal, and the snacks for each day, you will feel better and your body will get use to it. You must eat to lose. Just remember that it's how much you eat that counts.

Try this. See how it goes for you. Make up a menu for four weeks and prepare a different one each week. This will help you to be on your way.

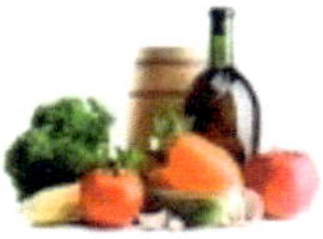

# Have Carrots, Will Travel

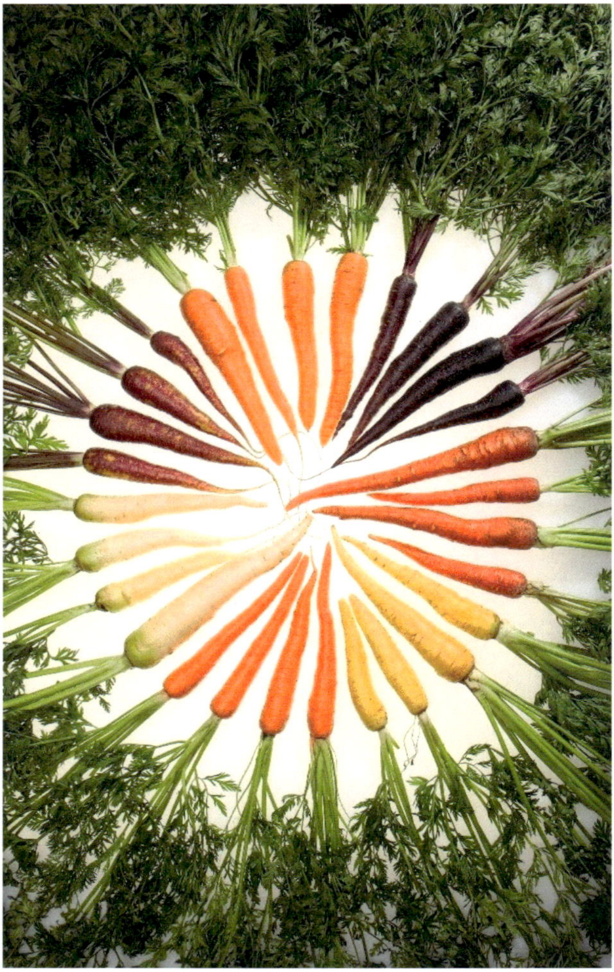

Chapter 7

# This Time, I Really Tried

You say that you really tried this time to lose weight. Right? Well go into your bedroom and get the pack of butter cookies from behind the headboard, and toss them in the trash. Go over to your sock drawer and get those peanut butter crackers, and put them in the trash with the cookies.

Now let's talk about trying. Before that, pick up that candy wrapper by your foot. Do you eat when you are by yourself? Do you only eat diet food when others are in the room? How many hands are up? I see a whole lot this time. Maybe we need a prayer to get back on the diet road. Hail to all of the thin people in the world. Don't throw your carrots at them. They can't help it because they are thin. Every calorie counts. They just don't know about that.

If you eat too many calories you will see fat piling up on you, but you know that by now. Somebody didn't throw a handful of fat at you and the fat just stuck on you. You had to work at it, right? You, can ask God to just remove the fat by Christmas. Don't forget the carrots, and celery. Watch to see when they are on sale. You can treat yourself to a nice salad, and a cold glass of ice tea with no sugar of course.

I munch on dry cornflakes and Graham Crackers. Those take the place of chips and cookies. Bet that blew your mind. What no chips? Now I won't make it. How are you going to feel when you lose your first ten pounds? The lost pounds will put a smile on your face, I'm sure. Never go shopping without bringing fresh fruit and vegetables home. Leave the chips and the cookies on the shelves. Don't start crying when you pass a shopping cart with all of the good stuff in it. Turn your head and go get some tuna and sugar-free jam. You can be thin by your next birthday.

We don't mess this up. Close your eyes and see yourself thinner. Now go and get a picture of yourself. Put it on the refrigerator. That will get your schedule back on the right road. Remember, don't tell anybody that you are on a diet. Let them tell you that you have lost some weight. You can shock the whole family with your weight-loss, and eat like a bird for the rest of our life - not really – just thought I would throw that in.

No wonder we get so big – every time you turn to another station, somebody is cooking some kind of a dish. We know how to cook. We could teach them a few dishes. We have to eat to live, but who wants to live until they are 105 years old? I didn't say to stop eating. Just don't eat as if it's your last supper. Take a breath.

Just think, when you lose your twenty pounds, you can help somebody else lose their weight. How proud will you be? Close your eyes and sit real still. Now can you see what you looked like about five years ago? Are you smiling yet? What a beauty right? Well every year God takes away a little more of our pretty looks. It's up to us to deal with what we have left. Take care of your face and hair. Don't let the wrinkles get the best of you.

I'm going to share my secret with you about wrinkles. Don't bury your face in the pillow when you sleep. Try to sleep on the corner of the pillow, and be sure your eyes aren't touching the pillow. This will help the bags under your eyes. Try it, and see for yourself.

Okay, how is it going with you lately? Are you getting out with your friends? Are you working on a hobby? Do you like crafts? Or, do you just eat every passing hour?

We must say a prayer and then do something about that real soon. Remember, God will help if you just ask and don't forget that He can see you when you are hiding with the brownie hanging out of your mouth. So the diet is still on. Have you bitten all of your nails down yet? Did you hurt the mailman or the neighbor? Well good, you are still in control. I will check on you in about two months from now. Hang in there.

My how time passes. You should have lost at least eight pounds by now. So you can feel better about yourself.

Dress up and go out. When someone says, "Oh, my you have really lost some weight. You look so nice," just smile and say, "Thank you." Now you know that you are on the right road and closer to your goal. Whatever you are doing, stay with it. Let others tell you that you have lost the weight. You may not feel the loss, but others can see the difference. A smaller size is on the way.

You can try to diet for a week. Then the second week, gets a little harder. By the time you lose a few pounds, you are so sick of celery and the carrots, you could die. Are you a person who can't go without sweets? We are in the same boat fishing for donuts. Do you have to have a cookie now and then, or a slice of cake with some milk?

So what are you going to do about this body? If you don't lose the weight, your knees will give out. Then you will walk like a duck. This is not a joke, and the pain is awful. Try getting up the stairs with a laundry basket. Then your knees will keep you up all night in pain. Please try and be good to yourself.

Look at all of the people who can't lose. Do you feel sorry for those who can't lose? Do you feel sorry for them? If everybody in the world was thin, we could wear the same clothes. I hope that everybody is thin in the next life. Just think, "No diets in Heaven!"

Clap your hands. Come to think of it, I never saw a picture of a fat angel. We need that angel with us all of the time, to fight off the diet devil. We can do this so put that piece of lunchmeat in the trash, and pick up a nice piece of baked fish.

You can only eat for so long. Time yourself. When did you start to eat? It should take about twenty minutes for a meal. If you are still stuffing the food in after twenty minutes, you were full ten minutes ago, but can't stop the fork from stuffing your face.

Get a grip on yourself and throw the darn fork in the trash. This diet is going to work and you are going to prove it. Eat the right foods, and drink plenty of water. Can you think of a better way to lose weight? If you know something that we don't know, pass it on. Remember that every diet is different. Some work, and some don't. I eat four small snacks a day - one meal with chicken and vegetables, and one meal that includes a fruit with a glass of tea or cold water. I don't seem to be so hungry, and it does fill me up. I snack on sliced peaches or an apple, or Graham Crackers, or dry cereal with no sugar. Try it and see what you think.

You have to eat small to get your body to burn the fat. If you don't eat, nothing will burn. It just kind of piles up. It's like a small fire. You have to throw a log on it once in a while to keep the fire from going out.

Don't ever go to bed hungry. Drink a little milk, or eat a few Graham Crackers. You will sleep a lot better. By the way, "Good night."

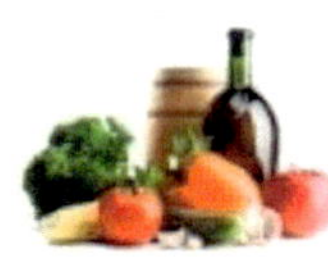

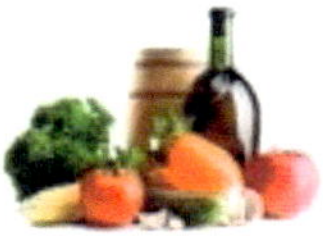

Chapter 8

# Let It All Hang Out

Notice the dieters that haven't quite lost enough weight yet. When they try on new clothes, the buttons don't seem to meet. The clothes look smaller than when they were on the hangers and the dieters think something is wrong with the mirror.

I have been there. How about you? I think that they are making the dressing rooms a bit smaller.

If you have tried more than five diets, and are still trying to lose the same weight, get down on your chubby little knees, and pray. Don't give up on yourself yet. You can still be saved. You can only say so much about diets, other than they stink worse than a rotten sack of potatoes. Throw out the potatoes, and get down to business.

Let's get back to the not-so-small body, and make it smaller. If you lift up your arm and see something wobble back and forth, it could be Mother Nature telling you to get off the couch and get going. Mother Nature does tricks on us, you know. When you get older, without any warning, you look into the mirror and see a face with a hanging bag under the left eye. You see wrinkles that look like a road map across your face, and you think "That can't be me – no way".

Your hips keep you up all night with pain and you always have to go to the bathroom about three (3:00 A.M.). You get out of bed and waddle to the bathroom. I thank God for all of my blessings. I'm just glad that when I go to the bathroom, both of my legs go at the same time. When I go into the kitchen, I'm just glad that I remember what I went in there for. This is not a trick. If you lose weight while you are young, remember that when you get older, it's in God's hands.

Make this your year to change your whole life, and think "diet". So take a chance and you will dance. So don't let it all hang out. Nobody wants to look at it.

Whenever you feel like giving up, find a picture of yourself when you gained the most weight, and put it in the kitchen. When you feel like stuffing your face, just take a good look at your picture. Believe me, you will stop in your tracks. Take a breath and reach for a can of tuna. Hang out with thin people once in a while. Watch the way they walk, the way they talk, how they dress, and then look at yourself.

Are you pleased with what you see? Now back to the diet. When you lose your weight, you will know how to walk, talk, and dress by being around the thin people. So who is helping who? The best day will come when you put your feet on the scale and you have lost twenty pounds.

Oh, my God, you did it. I am so proud of you. Now you need to go and buy a new outfit to show off your "new you". So now you can let it all hang out and strut your stuff. Go girl and let those donuts and cookies know who is the boss. Have carrots and celery will travel.

I'm going to say a prayer for all those who are really trying real hard. I'm going to ask God to step in and help them to reach their goal. Diets are not fun, but the payoff is great. You can have a friend or a family member participate in a diet with you. Set a goal for four months and see who will lose the most weight. You know that there will be only one winner, but the loser will not really be a loser. They will have lost weight too.

I see nice thin women, and wonder what they eat. Do they walk a lot? Do they eat like a bird? I know a couple of women who eat large amounts of anything they want. They always dress nicely and look so trim. Please God, what is their magic?

There are a lot of other women who sure would like to know that answer. To know would be a blessing all in one. Do you ever think that your middle name is diet? Do you always get interested when you see an ad for a new diet? You keep looking for the "one" that will work for you. After about a few months on a diet you just get so sick. You just want to cry.

Okay, have your cry, and then let's get thin. Some days are not too bad, and some days are a cry for help. The best thing of the day is taking off your bra and getting a good night's rest.

Good night to all of the dandy dieters, and may God bless you with thinner hips.

Some ideas to help you along is if you are having a hard time getting started, get a cookbook and just sit and look at the pictures for a while, but not in the kitchen. Are you getting full yet? Don't look at the brownies, or the cookbook will fly. Look at the food and get some ideas on shopping for more fruits and greens. Fiber will help you in a big way. Don't forget Graham Crackers. They are a life saver.

You can relax and do this by Christmas. This will be your present from the Lord, Himself. Come on now, don't think this is all hog wash. Do you like it when you sit on a chair and the chair disappears; or when you bend over to pick something up, you come up with purple lipstick and red blotches on your face? How does it feel when you have an itch on your foot, and you can't even reach it to scratch.

This book is for anybody who wants to get in better shape and feel better about themselves. When you start to lose weight, don't forget to tell your friends about this magical book. They just may need a good laugh.

Do you remember the last time you turned down any food and what it was? Notice that after a while, you didn't even miss it? Do that for about five months, and then count all of the calories that you saved your body from burning. Your body will thank you, I'm sure.

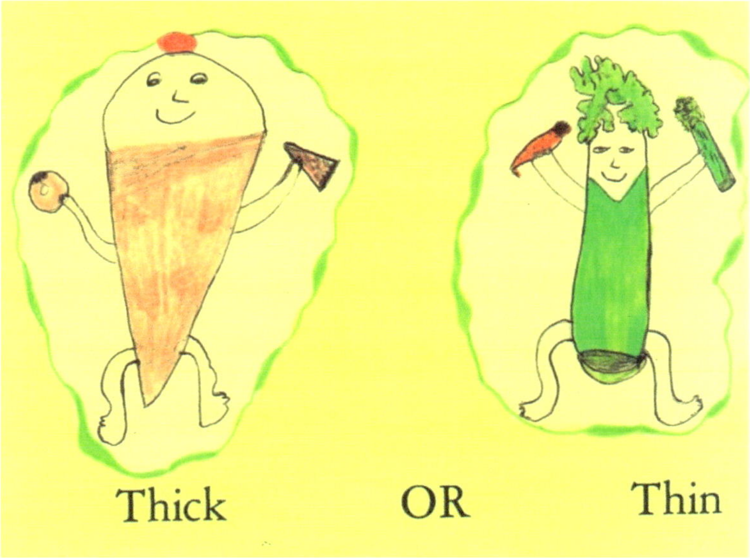


Judith Schwartz, artist

So what will it be – thick or thin? Take your pick. I know that all dieters want to be thin, but you have to earn it with hard work. God didn't say it was going to be easy, and He sure was right.

Do you remember some of the people with whom you went to school? You see them now and they are about fifty pounds heavier than they were in school. You remember the girl that was real heavy and had a hard time trying to lose weight? Well guess what? She is now thin and a good dresser. All of the spots on her face are gone. So guess who is a real knock-out? Is that girl you or somebody you wanted to be? I could have written about birds or flowers, but I thought it would be better if I could help you to lose weight, and to keep you from wearing that paper, cold gown in the doctor's office.

If you lose ten pounds from reading this book, that's ten pounds that your body doesn't have to carry around anymore. The idea is to lose the weight so you don't have anything to hang out – not a pretty picture.

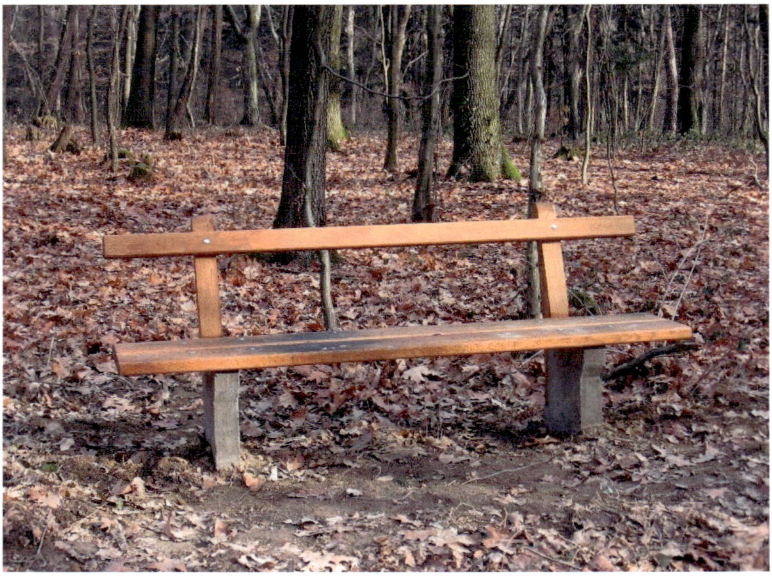

Photo by Mimica, www.Rgbstock.com

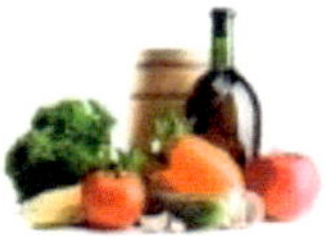

Chapter 9

# Being Over-Weight is Not Fun

Being heavy is not funny at all. We see large people all the time. They try to diet but they just get depressed. Yes, this is a problem for a lot of good people in the world. Some of us just can't lose no matter what we do. We hate it when we can't eat what we like. Sometimes it puts us in a bad mood, and makes it hard for us to get along with others.

Thin people could never feel our pain. They never had to do so. They have a pain of their own. I think it is so rude to make fun of a heavy person. They didn't ask to be that way. They were not blessed with trim legs and a thin body.

It's not easy for thin people because maybe they would like to have a few pounds. So let's bless them with some. Thin people are more active and are blessed by far. They can eat anything they want and still stay the same. I would like that for sure. How about you? Thin people run. They work out and do exercises. So let's give them a hand. It's not easy for them either. They have to work out all of the time because they want to feel good. Let's lose weight and give them a run for their slim shape

Now if you lose six pounds, don't go crazy and have some cookies or ice cream. Okay? We see a lot of celebrities that are heavy and they are famous. You're thinking, "Well they have the money to help them along." You may be right, but don't you think that some are not satisfied with the way they look, and have the same problem that we do? You can have all the money in the world and still have a weight problem. We know that we are not rich but we can still make choices. We can be thin if that's what we really want.

I know you get depressed and tired of eating the same old stuff. Try new ideas. Look in cookbooks for foods that are low fat and low in sugar. Some aren't bad at all. My friend always eats popcorn. It fills her up and keeps her from eating sweets. So how many Dandy Dieters do we have with big eyes, short fingernails, and a nervous condition? I thought so. That's why they call us "dandy" because we are special. We will be thin to prove it.

Have you heard anybody talking about a thin person lately? Then why do they talk about heavy people? Heavy people try to dress the best way they can. I saw a thin girl at the store the other day. She was so sloppy. Her shoes and clothes were dirty. Her hair was messy. But guess what, she was built so nicely. I thought, "If I were built like her, I sure would look better."

Maybe she lost her job, and is doing the best that she can. But that just goes to show you, you can have everything and still have problems. We have to believe that we can do this dieting because we do have trouble with our weight. You can get depressed, cry and be mad, but when you wipe your tears, you are still heavy. Did you ever go to the store and ask the butcher to weigh one pound of fat and put it in a plastic wrap? Well I did. It worked for a while. Every time I would go to eat, I would look at the big ball of fat. Someone could get thin real fast, and I did. Then I tossed the fat in the trash, and it was over. Try it sometime. You wouldn't believe what a pound of fat looks like.

Fat is not funny, and it never was. So how many of us are going to be thin next year? Do I have any hands up? Take a breath. Say a prayer. The thin people won't know you when you pass them on the street. Did you ever say, "I'm going to lose twenty pounds before Easter, Christmas, or my birthday"? I'm sure you did, but how many times did you say that? Those days have come and gone. Yet your large belly and legs are still following you around in the store.

While writing this book, at times I got what they call writers' block. I wonder if you can get a diet block. We just have to locate the problem and work on it, and show the "No, No List" who is the boss.

We have to get off the couch and turn the tube off. Get in an exercise class or just do some exercises at home to get your body used to the routines. Start off slowly and don't throw your left leg up over your head. You just might have a purple face and a broken leg. Check with your insurance to see what injury they will cover.

Is it time for a break yet? Meet me back here in five minutes. I have to get a "small" apple and a glass of "skim" milk. Are you back yet? Get out of that kitchen and put that peanut butter and those crackers back. Who do you think I'm writing this book for – a real skinny person?

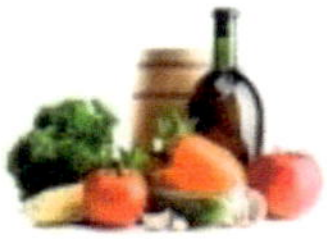

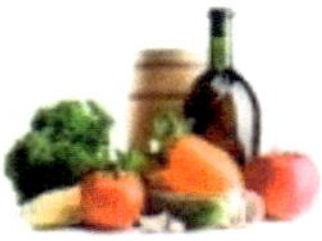

Chapter 10

# Diet 'Til You Die

How many of you have been on a diet from the time your Mom put on your baby shoes? Okay, if Mom couldn't help you and you can't help yourself, what is the next step? Are we going to diet for the rest of our lives? If we can't get thin while we are alive, then maybe we will look good when we die.

Okay, but I would like to be thin so I can enjoy a thin life. How about you? You can go to a gym, walk with friends, swim at the beach... What are you doing to help yourself? Nobody can help you, but you! Why would you want to give up on a great person as yourself? You don't have to diet 'til you die.

You need to find a better way to eat, such as less food and the right food. Don't eat just because it's lunch time, but eat only when you are hungry.

Try not to eat the same food all of the time. Eat fruits. Everybody likes watermelon and strawberries. If you don't, eat what you like.

Exercise will help you to stay on the right track. When you reach your goal, God will give you a rainbow. I have written this book for all those who cheat on a diet. "Hello, are you there?" You with the cookie hanging out of your mouth - do you eat like a bird in front of everybody? Then do you eat like three people when you are alone? So what's going on upstairs or in the stomach?

Don't be so hard on yourself. If you eat the wrong things, just try a little harder. You can't fall off of the floor. You are already down, so pick yourself up and make a fresh start. You are still the same person. You just want to be a thinner person. So spit out that cookie. Remember, my dear diet cheater, if you cheat, you pay the price, and you can't pay in cookies.

You don't have to diet 'til you die. You just have to work on a different way to eat. For all those who have stocks in fast foods, go to the fast food company of your choice. Buy the hamburger that is bothering you. Smell it. Then throw it as far as you can. Now that's fast food. Do you feel any better?

Not all people are born to be heavy. God gave us a smart mind, but we make the choices. We eat too many calories and eat when we are depressed. The food will make you feel better but it won't take away the problem. If you try to get rid of the problem first, then you won't eat so much. You will have so many things to do, you won't even think about eating.

I know a girl who has been trying to lose twenty-five pounds for about ten years. Do you know of a friend in the same boat? Is it you? It's not so easy. Is it? We all have days like that. We must get a hobby. I don't mean counting chips, and Long John pastries.

Try counting slices of apples. I do know that apples are good for you. They fill you up. If you can stay on a diet longer than four weeks, come the following Saturday, you can celebrate by having a cold beer, and some cookies. Does that sound good, or what?

Once in a while you can have a small bite of the good stuff, just to keep you alive, but don't overdo it. It's hard to go to a BBQ when you are on a diet. You have to think, "Are those baby-back-ribs better than being thinner?" I know at that time, the ribs will win. You can make up for it the next day, so enjoy yourself, and have a nice day with your friends. I hope that you have a great time at the BBQ.

Now back to the nasty diet. You know what that means. You don't have to count calories, if you don't want to do so. I think the trick to this madness is just to eat small. If you learn how to eat the right foods, then after a while, dieting won't even bother you.

I just know that you would like to throw a box of donuts at me about now. Go ahead. I haven't had a good donut in sometime. I won't bluff you, you do have to stay away from the high-calorie foods. I think donuts are on the top of the list, next to that slice of pizza you are getting ready to shove into your mouth.

Please don't eat like a truck driver while you are reading this book. If you do, a prayer won't even help you. What is our next holiday? Now set a goal to lose about ten pounds. That will put you into a real nice outfit to show off the new you. Don't you feel a lot better about yourself, when you look into the mirror? See yourself getting thinner, and know that God is on our side.

You are a very special person. You can do things that other people can't do. Don't give up on yourself. Why would you put great value on something, and not value yourself? YOU CAN DO IT.

Now close your eyes, and in your mind, can you see yourself and how you looked back ten years ago? Were you thinner then? Was your hair the same color? How do you feel about the way you were dressed? Do you have a smile on your face? Is it a sad look? Now baby, it's time to get in shape and keep that smile for life. Doesn't that feel better?

Now, let's say we are on the second week of the diet. How is it going? Do we want to jump into a bag of potato chips? Are we hiding cookies under our pillow at night? You can have all of the hiding places to stash your goodies, but you will have to carry around the fat after you eat them.

Look down at one side of the chair where you are sitting. If you see a hang-over, throw the good stuff in the ditch, and keep going. I get so tired of being on a diet. I want to go and check out the good stuff in the ditch. How about you? Have you ever seen a fat ditch?

God, please bless my fat. I know right where it's at. Isn't it strange that we can really try to lose weight and feel like the scale is just not moving? Then you go to the store and run into a friend or two. They say, "Boy have you lost the weight." You can't buy that feeling with money. It will make you feel so good. It should, because you have been giving up the good stuff for someone to notice you. They did.

This is not an easy thing to do. Yes, I would like to eat some pizza and a burger and onion rings. But, I traded them in for a few Graham Crackers, and skim milk. I know you are saying, "Go girl! I'm on my way to the fast food place for lunch."

That's okay with me. I'm going to be thin by Christmas, and you are going to be looking for something to wear. You can tell me how good your hamburger was.

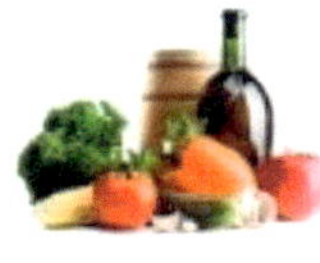

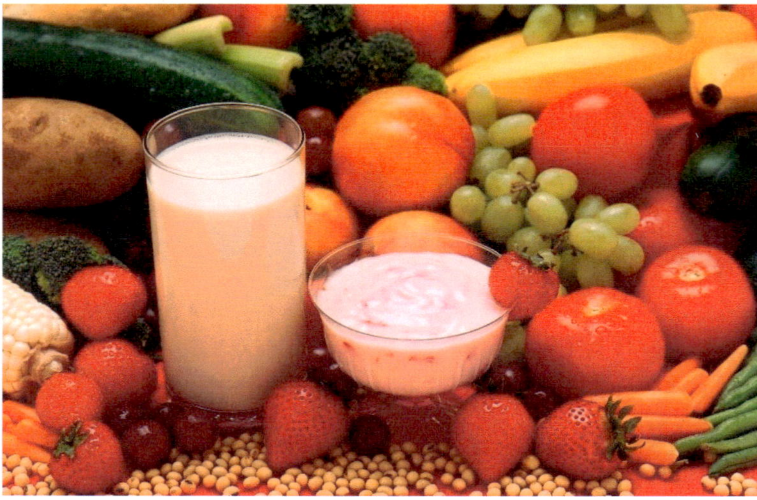

If you can go for two months on a good diet, you will be saved. You say that you have only lost sixteen pounds? Well think of it this way, if for some reason you pass away on the diet, you will sure look a little thinner while your family is staring at you. By the way, I'm glad I met you.

---

# Have Carrots And Celery Will Travel

Chapter 11

# Have Carrots and Celery Will Travel

Let's face it, nobody can eat carrots and celery for the rest of their life, unless you have hair growing between your toes. We need to have protein for sure. Don't forget all of those good vitamins.

Now take a deep breath and read on. I will get to the good stuff. A diet is hard enough on our nerves right? I can't get through a week without those little things with a hole in it. Come on, we all know what donuts taste like. Don't we? Just look at those extra-large buns we are sitting on. Well, another good donut goes in the ditch. Right?

Let's move on to another sad diet day. We have to make up our minds first that we are going to do this right. I have tried everything I know, and I think that I lost the same ten pounds 30 times in my life-time.

What is the trick for keeping it off? If you know, please e-mail me via "nofatinheaven@thankGod.com"

If you feel real heavy when you walk, you are carrying around three two-year olds, you can't see them but you can feel their weight.

There are reasons how you know that your name is at the top of the diet list.

- When you are walking to your car and you feel like you have two bricks in your shoes that should give you a big hint.
- When you drop your pen, you bend over to pick it up, and all of a sudden, you can't breathe, this is due to the large hump around your mid-section.
- When you go to the store, if you can't race over to the table with the cakes on sale, you must go on a diet.

That tells me that your diet list is on the table under the pile of papers, and you haven't seen it for some time. If you are thinking of an excuse, save it for a real dumb person. Now onto the carrots and celery. You can munch on them, and they will fill you up and not out as chips and dip. They may not taste as good, but the carrots and celery will get you closer to your weight goal.

Is it time for a break? Go and get yourself some carrots and wave them to the thin people. Have Carrots and Celery Will Travel. May God bless our large bodies, before we lose the weight.

Do you have any good ideas on how to lose a few pounds? Please pass the tips on for I'm sure the rest of us would like some hints and a prayer.

I think my back goes out more than I do and my stomach gets there before the rest of me does. I have been on so many diets until I thought that someday I might write a book on the darn fat, and get it over with. How am I doing?

Let's have a little test. Only you will know the right answers. Okay, here goes. How would you grade yourself from 1 to 10? Be honest with yourself. If your score is over sixty, there is no hope. Sorry!

1. Are you heavy because you are unhappy?
2. Do you eat just to be eating, and you are not really hungry?
3. Are you bored and have no hobbies?
4. Do you eat out of depression?
5. Are you lonely?
6. Do you have too much time on your hands?
7. Do you shop when you are hungry?
8. Must you eat sweets every day?
9. Do your children make you want to eat?
10. Is your spouse having an affair?
11. Are you getting a divorce?
12. Are you dealing with drugs, or booze?
13. Do you have an illness?
14. Are you unemployed, and can't get a job?

Any of these can be the problem. I pray that God will help you along the way, because you are a special person. If you know what the problem is and you are at work trying to get rid of it, you will take some of the weight off your shoulders.

There is a “better YOU” waiting to be seen by others. So let’s make it happen. You can be sad all of your life, but you can make yourself happy too. Get a new hairdo. Be around others who are trying to lose weight too. Exchange recipes. Now let’s see who can lose ten pounds first. After a while, it does get better. You don’t even miss some of the foods that made you heavy in the first place. God, please answer our prayers.

There are many reasons why we are heavy. Only you know what your reasons are. Mine is sugar. I love cookies and other sweets. I would pass up meat, and potatoes for a good donut, and a cup of coffee. Now I am trying to get to the next day without any sweets. It’s in God’s hands.

You don’t have to count calories all day. Just think before you stuff your face with food. Take a breath. Eat on a smaller plate. Eat half of a sandwich, and drink ice water instead of soda. Try wheat crackers instead of chips. Munch on fruit, or veggies instead on junk food. So if you try this for about a month, maybe your body will get the message.

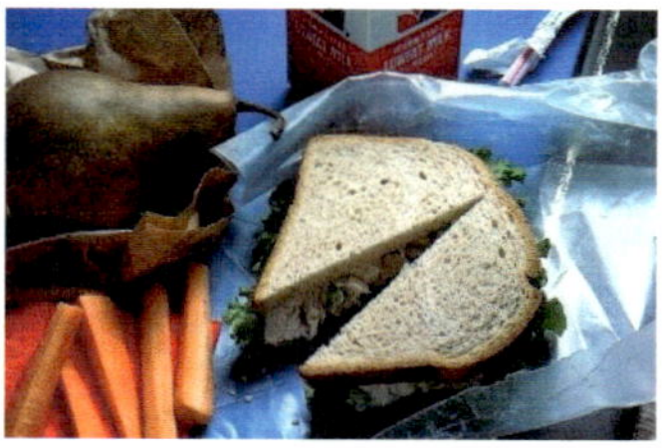

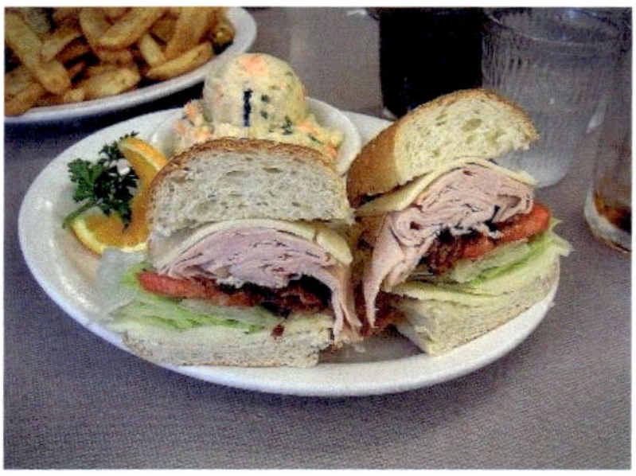

Now close your eyes and let's say a food prayer.

**Dear Lord,**

Please sit at the table while I eat my meal. I hope that when my body has had enough, you will knock my plate on the floor. Please Lord, help me every day to eat the right food that will make my behind smaller. Amen.

Now if we say that prayer, now and then, it just might help. So what do you say? Are there any heavy-weights out there that want to be thin for the next holiday, and walk through the door with your head up high instead of walking with thick thighs?

Bet that made you smile a little. Then, drop that candy bar. Don't tell anybody that you are on a diet. They will look at you too closely to see if you have lost any weight. That could make you crazy. May God go with you and your diet.

I went shopping the other day. I went into the store, got a basket and went right past the table with cookies and pies on it. Before I realized it, I was getting a head of lettuce. I felt pretty good, and I didn't feel as if I was on a diet.

I think that after a while, you just adjust to the circumstance, and it doesn't bother you. God heard my prayer, and I will not give up on myself. Don't think that there is no hope for you, because there is. It doesn't matter how old you are. Remember Judy's mom. If my Mom can lose weight at eighty-eight, anybody can. As for me, I'm still trying.

When I am on the computer, I snack on green peppers and they don't taste too badly. The other day, my husband said to me, "What is that stuff on your face?" I said, "That is my wrinkle cream. I'm waiting for it to take effect." While you are trying to lose weight, you can work on your face. Every little bit helps.

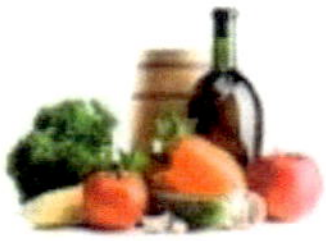

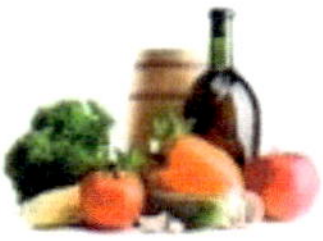

Chapter 12

# Be A Busy Body

We like nice clothes. We want our hair to look nice. We want our bodies to be thinner. Do I have any dreamers? Let's try this time and make that dream come true. Your whole life will change with a new you. It doesn't matter how old you are. My Mom would not eat bread and sweets for two weeks. She then dropped six pounds. As I told you, she is eighty-eight years old. God, I hope that she doesn't read this book because I just told the world how old she was.

But you see, Mom always kept busy. She use to paint the house, sew doll clothes, make wedding dresses and veils, and still get the supper on the table at five (5:00 P.M.). She made home-made biscuits, and cheese noodles. If you are on a diet, don't go to Mom's house for Thanksgiving. I warned you.

This is the time to be a busy body. Keep your mind off food, but not MOM's. If you don't lose any weight, I don't want to hear about your broken scale. Throw it in the trash and buy a new one. Maybe it's not so bad to be a busy body. Just work on yourself, and the reward will be out of sight.

I like the friends that are always telling us what to eat. Notice that they could be eating the same thing. They should look in the mirror before they give advice. However, maybe your friends would like to have you around for a while. They just want you to be healthy. That's not a busy body. That's a caring friend.

How busy was your body today? Did you exercise, or take a walk? Every little bit helps. Time for a break. Go and get some coffee and some Graham Crackers. I'll meet you back here in ten minutes.

Coffee break is over. Now put that piece of chicken in the trash. No eating after seven (7:00 P.M.) Drink some tea or some skim milk. Remember, don't be a busy body, but keep your body busy. Have carrots and celery will travel. Think like a rabbit.

A busy body can help a senior. Take them to the store, or take them out to lunch. I'm sure they would like that. Work part-time in an office. Be around people who need your service. Your mind won't be on food if you keep it busy.

Weight can hold us back. It's so hard on our knees. The knees will keep you up all night in pain. How is the old back holding out? Think of all the times you went to the doctor for the pain. Maybe if we lost about twenty pounds, our backs would say "Thank you, baby."

Was there anything that you read that was of any help? I hope so. You will feel better about yourself when you lose some weight. You have to like yourself, first to reach your goal. Doesn't success feel good?

I know that you can do it. Next time you go to the doctor's office, you can get on the scale with a smile and surprise them. Don't you just hate to get on that scale and hear how much you have gained? So don't be depressed. Get dressed in a smaller size.

Did you ever get on a bus and feel that the seats were made smaller? Maybe our behinds are getting a bit larger from the "It won't hurt to stop at the fast food for that double hamburger." Need I say more? There are many reasons why it is so hard to lose weight. Some people have no problem at all while others feel it is a "no win" deal.

Medicine also contributes to weight-gain. You will hold water from taking medicine, and it will be very hard to lose weight. This can't be helped. I'm sure some of you know that's right. We have to think thin and keep busy. Someday, we will be able to remove our big clothes, and replace them with smaller ones.

When you lose the weight, you can help others that are having no luck with their weight-loss. Everybody needs a little push now and then to get going. This book is your push. Read it, and pass it on to someone who needs to read it. Everybody is different in the way they lose weight. If it's hard for you, just keep doing what you are doing, and in time it will happen. Don't give up on yourself.

When was the last time that you got dressed up and went out to a real nice place? Why are the nice clothes still hanging on hangers? For whom are you saving them? Do you think they will like the same style? Let's hang up smaller sizes on the hangers. May God bless our new clothes on the way to our hangers. I know it's in God's hands.

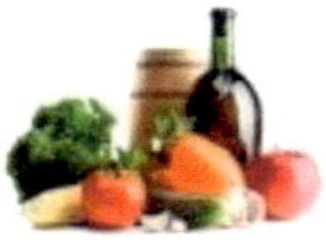

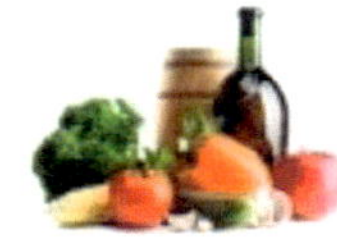

Chapter 13

# Help For The Thin

I know there are thin people who are having a hard time trying to gain a few pounds. Oh please, let us help you. I also know there are a lot of readers who are waving their carrots in the air. We know what not to eat to lose the weight, but how can we help the thin people? Is there anybody out there who would like to help the “little” people?

I don’t mean the people who have been on a diet for nine months. Somebody could get hurt real bad, you know. It’s not hard to gain weight. Just ask all of us junk food eaters.

For starters, if you need to gain weight, eat a few donuts with a cup of coffee. God, I’m getting hungry already. First you can eat a ham sandwich with lettuce, tomato and Mayo on white bread. Have some chips with onion dip and a soda with a bowl of strawberry ice cream. I can hardly take this anymore.

How are all of you dieters doing out there? Are you trying to move the refrigerator into your bedroom? Take a breath and get a grip on yourself. Think “thin”.

If you are a thin person and wonder why some people can’t lose weight, then why can’t you gain any? That works both ways. We just want to help you while we are trying to help ourselves.

If you are trying to gain a few pounds, try eating some cookies with milk and don't forget the pizza that is on everybody's mind. You should have gained at least four pounds by now. So how are you doing? Are your clothes a bit tight and do you look a little fuller? Glad we could help. We love to share. I can always find somebody to help you.

Thin people want to feel good about themselves too. Some people are a little too thin and just can't gain any weight. Yet they eat like a truck driver. All of us who are walking to one side would like to have your problem on our "to do list". I can think of so many people who would like to hit the thin people in the head with their carrots. Stand in line. May God hold back all of the "Dandy Dieters".

Why do you think that heavy people always have a smile on their face when they see a nice dressed thin person? It's because they are wanting to be that person more than anything. They are so tired of being on a diet. Sometimes they don't even bother to eat at all.

I wonder, do the thin people ever get heavy as they get older? The hardest thing to do is when you have to buy a larger size, because you can't get that extra-large leg into the slacks you have been wearing for the past three years.

Thin people don't ever have to worry about that one. Down, you starving dieters. Eat another carrot. It's break time. You go to the bathroom and get some skim milk. Meet me back here in five minutes.

I'm back. Now where are you? Get out of those crackers and put that jelly back. I said to go to the bathroom, not to fill up until you can't take another bite.

If thin people would help heavy people to lose weight, then maybe the dieters wouldn't have it so hard. This would encourage the dieters when they see a nice dress that they like, or a nice outfit they wish that they could wear. Make that wish come true. With prayer, you can do it.

Sincerely, thin people gain weight for the same reason as heavy people who want to lose. They want to feel better about themselves. What dieter in the whole world can say that it's easy to lose weight? There are none that I know. How many times have you sat and cried because you are so heavy and wanted to eat whatever you desired? If you could eat anything you wanted right now, what would it be?

Can you taste the flavor as you chew? Does it taste real good? Now wake up. The dream is over. Down to business, and get the good thoughts out of your mind. The ditch must be pretty full by now, and still more good stuff to come.

You don't have to carry carrots around for the rest of your life. You can share them with the thin people. How do you know? They just might like them. The next time I see you at the store, I hope that you are a little lighter, and that I have lost at least fifteen pounds. What a blessing!

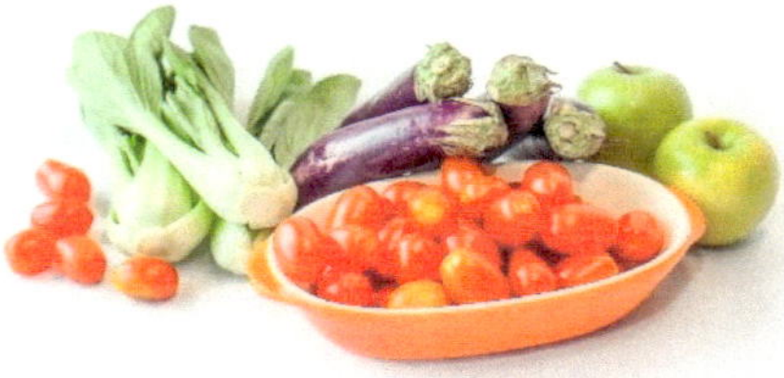

If you can stand up and look down, and see your feet without losing your breath, hang on to that diet. It's working, baby. Keep up the good work. Have carrots will travel, and have body will get better. Yes, it's in God's hands.

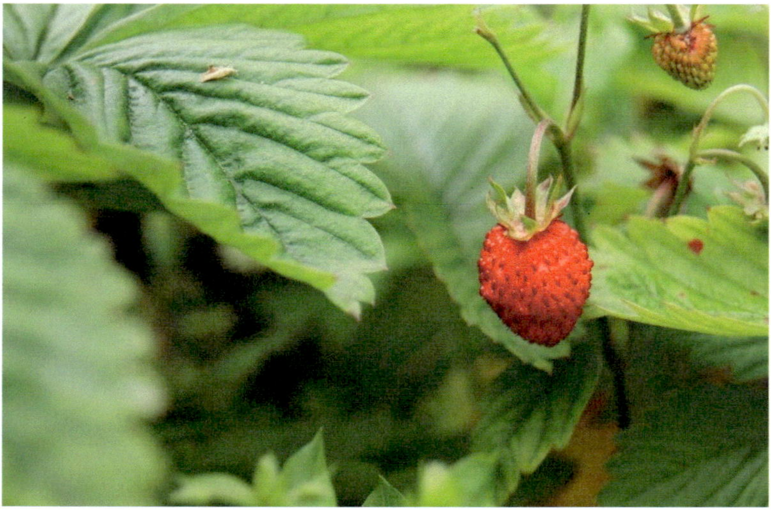

Photo by AL71, www.Rgbstock.com (strawberries)

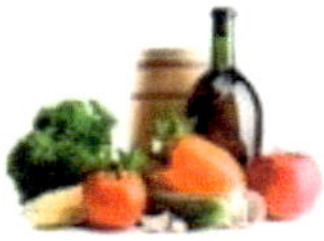

Chapter 14

# Belly-Up

Your nervous system is on cruise control after ten months of being on a diet. Nobody got hurt and your hunger pains are at peace. How proud you are when people tell you how nice you look. They ask you how much weight have you lost, but they don't know of the struggle you went through to get where you are. At times when you're not eating pizza for so long, you could have made a neighbor disappear. You can rearrange the furniture so many times. The diet seems to be getting a little better, and you can now see yourself getting thinner.

Your face looks thinner, and your nose comes to a point, but your belly is still the same, and the hump is not moving. This might take some real courage to get rid of the belly-up.

I know a girl who was on a diet for four months, and lost twenty-five pounds. She looked so nice and you could see that her face was thinner, and her behind was smaller, but her belly-up was still there. It's like she lost weight all around her body, but her stomach didn't move.

What are we to do, lay on the floor and throw our legs up over our heads, and hope that we don't pass out, or roll on the floor like a fish out of water? If you are still on the diet when you get older, remember that you are not over the hill. You're just too tired to climb the hill.

If you are eighty or older, throw the diet in the trash and pig out, but keep "healthy" in mind. If you are lucky to live past eighty, you can eat anything you want. I'm sure you will never forget your life-time of diets.

Diets are no fun. It's like trying to back out of a bad marriage. How many out there are belly-up – can't get rid of the darn thing no matter what you do? Like I said before, you can cry about it but it won't help until you make up your mind and do something about it. God never forgot about you. He will be with you all the way. If you find the right diet for you, and your belly falls off, just step over and keep going.

Do you know any way to lose the belly-up? Please share it with us so our belly don't touch the wheel when we drive the car. I like more room between me and the wheel. After all, I'm driving, not my belly. I did think of a girdle but then I thought, "Why should I be heavy and miserable?" So there is the belly-up blocking the view of my feet when I stand up. That's okay, I can see them when I sit down.

It's break time for all those dieters in control. Are you in control? Then meet me back here in ten minutes.

I'm back. Where are you? Spit that cookie out of your mouth, and put that soda back. You can pick on cucumbers. They hit the spot. When you lost about twenty pounds, did you notice that everything was at a stand-still? You have to just keep doing what you are doing until the body starts up again.

Don't start eating a little here, and a little there. The next time that you weigh yourself, you will be shocked at how fast the weight piles back. I have been on a diet for three months now. I don't count calories. I'm just eating as I want to eat for the rest of my life. I can tell from how I feel that I think this is the best way to lose weight. I don't act as if I'm on a diet. I don't buy anything with a lot of sugar such as cookies. Juices also have a lot of sugar in them.

I changed from high calorie foods to diet foods and to low-calorie foods. You can save a lot of calories and as time goes by, it doesn't even bother you. You eat half of what you were use to eating. If you want a chip, eat two and go on your way. If you can do that, you are showing the diet who's the boss. I have seen people go on a diet, and lose up to forty pounds. The next time you see them they have gained all of their weight back. They do fast weight-loss diets and their body is in shock until they start back eating the junk food again. Hello fat, here I am.

I was told that if you lose weight in a short time, it will come back by your next birthday. Lose the weight slowly and longer. Your body can adjust to a set eating pattern. In time, your body will start dropping weight. I'm still waiting for you to get off the couch, and get down to business. How about it "thunder thighs"?

Remember that we still have to deal with the belly-up. So put on your seat belt. You're on a mission of many miles. See you when you get back. Good luck!

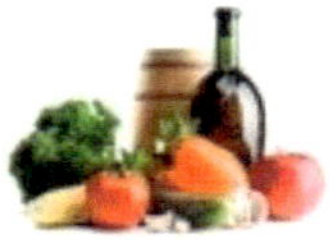

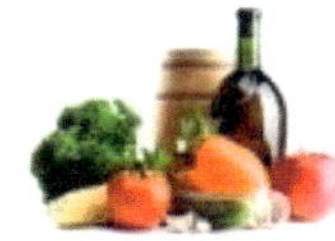

Chapter 15

# Diet Devil On Duty

Did you hear that loud noise? It's the diet devil sitting on your right shoulder laughing his head off because you are eating a jelly donut. He knows that he has put some diet evil in you. Enjoy your donut then drag those large hips around for the rest of your life. Did I get your attention?

What is going on with you? Why are you stuffing your mouth with anything you can get in your hands? Have you lost your mind? This is about fat or defeat. Take your pick. You might as well go to the thrift store and buy the biggest pair of pants that you can find. Forget about "thinner by Christmas".

How long have you been carrying around the diet devil and eating like there are three hundred Thanksgiving days a year. You can start by knocking that diet devil off of your shoulder and don't worry if he bangs his head. Get your head clear. Say a prayer. Then get a glass of water and a carrot. Ask the diet Angel to protect you. Do you have your seat belt on yet? Are you ready to ride down the road to a thinner body? Okay, let's go big gal and check out that outfit you are going to get into by Christmas. You have to be on guard and watch out for the diet devil. He will come at you with a pizza and some chips. He will try to put diet evil into you again. So beware.

I'm sure you are big enough to fight him off. He is always on duty looking for dieters who can't control their fork and they think meal time lasts for forty minutes. When you reach your goal, the diet angel should be sleeping on your shoulder and the diet devil will be looking for a strange person on a diet.

This is a fight. Your business is to lose weight. You have to fight off the food, the diet devil and your enemies that want you to gain instead of lose. Keep your seat belt on and drive a little faster, but don't get a ticket. They cost money.

Did you make up your mind yet? Do you need a little help to really be on your last diet – forever? You always heard that you have never walked in my shoes. Well, this diet better work, or you will be singing, "You have never walked in my clothes."

The diet devil is watching you eat that piece of pound cake. That's the way to go happy hips! What are you doing? Do you think you are at happy hour with the diet devil? So waddle yourself out of there and get yourself together. You have a lot of work to do, lamb chops.

Remember if your diet doesn't work, you can't go to the body shop and buy a smaller behind.

You have to eat small to be small. Did you get that? Or should I put it in large print to get your attention? By the way, how was your pound cake? I'm talking to that bulge hiding under your blouse.

Let's get down to business. Make up a new diet menu. There are real good diet dishes that can help your hunger and keep you on the right track. My favorite is strawberry Jell-O, yogurt, and blackberries. Try this and enjoy. Put your body first in life. Your body will have a long life. That came out pretty good.

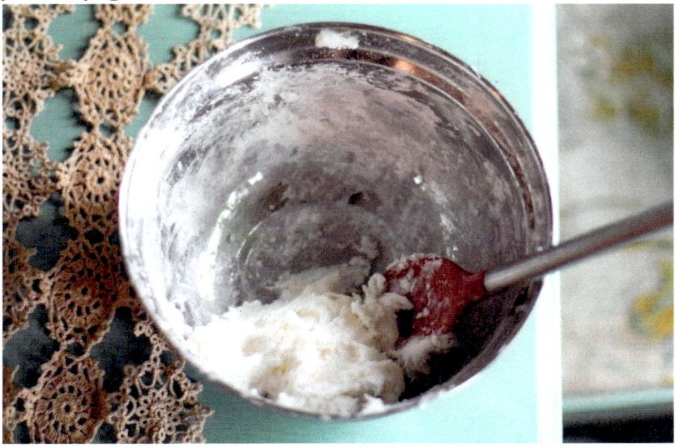

You can always hide your big feet in a pair of shoes, but try hiding your belly under a nice blouse. You can see the hump way across the room. Doesn't that make you want to lose weight or what? What happened to "have carrots, will travel"? Did you trade your carrots for pizza and cake? By Christmas, your face will be so full, you will look like you had Botox. We don't want to scare Santa, do we?

Call me when you lose ten pounds, and we will celebrate with a nice sub sandwich. They are so darn good. If you can think of an easier way to lose weight, please don't keep it a secret. Tell us about the magic. You seem to be doing a little better now. Did you send the diet devil on his way? He will be back, so watch out.

When you lose weight, and start to feel good, your whole attitude will change. But when you gain some back, don't you feel as if a boat came in, and has a leak in it? You can always put a carrot in the hole.

I smell BBQ. Don't you see the diet devil sitting on the window ledge? He is waiting for you to run for the pit. Turn around and run the other way. Let him eat your half. Wait a minute. Where are you going? Grab a piece of fruit and get going. You have two months to lose weight before Christmas. This just may be your present from Santa. So keep your pork roast on the diet, and really surprise the whole family when you come through the door.

I see that the diet devil is working on you again. Push him off of your shoulder and show him who the boss is. If he was smart, he would go to the gym. There are plenty of shoulders to ride on and discourage the dieters. Keep eating those carrots and cucumbers, and trade those large legs in for a pair of thin thighs. I hope that I'm not too hard on you. I just want you to look real nice for the holiday in that green outfit with the red trim.

You can take your car in for body work, but you have to work on your own human body, so the parts will look good. What's more important – to have a nice car, or to ride in a car with a dent, and have a real nice body? Everything is going up - gas, food, bills, taxes, and our hips waving in the air.

Let's lose the weight and be in better health. Your doctor will wonder where you are. Get a large box. Put all of your big clothes in it, and only hang up clothes that you want to get into. You can always get something out of the box if things don't work out.

A diet is only a way of life. Don't let it control you. Be tough. You better get busy. I see the diet devil coming your way. Get out the grapes and strawberries, and maybe he will leave. You have to be on guard at all times, or he will wave a slice of pizza in your face. He will do anything to help you gain more weight.

It's break time. You go and get an orange. Meet me back here in five minutes.

I hear you in there. What are you doing? Get back here. We have to talk about diets and thinner bodies. So how are you doing so far? I hope that I could help you to feel better about yourself and to really lose some weight. I didn't write this book to hurt anyone – only to help them. I'm in the same boat as you. I think my boat has a leak in it. If you are having a hard time losing weight, don't give up, and say you can't do it. There is a way that you can do it.

Move around more and eat less. When you put food on your plate, just put a little of each thing. Say to yourself that you can always get more. After a while, you can't even eat the little bit you have on your plate. In time, your body will be satisfied with the smaller amounts, and you will be on your way to thin city. I hope the very best for you. GOOD LUCK!

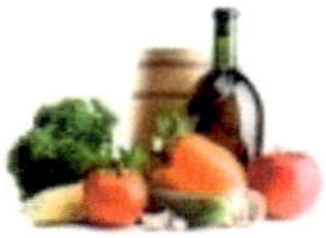

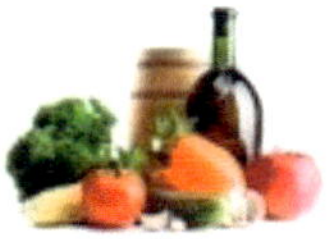

Chapter 16

# Help Is On The Way

Are you tired of everybody trying to tell you how to lose weight? You can add me to the list. I guess if God wants me to have this body, I'm going to help you lose weight. At least one of us will be thin. This is a test where you can't see your grade until you reach your goal.

Like any other test, you must work on it. So bring out the lettuce and the tomatoes. Forget about the diet devil for a while. He's at a diet class waiting for a dieter to come out so he can jump on her shoulder.

We all lose weight in different ways and try diets and then gain the weight back. This time it's going to work. If I can help you lose some weight, and feel better about yourself, that will be my reward.

I don't know all of the answers. If I did, I would be blowing the dust around the dance floor about now. Like I said, "Help is on the way". Try some of these menus. They will fill you up and taste pretty good. You can eat pizza, chips, and cookies. It's more so of how much you eat, and how you eat.

Let's take pizza. You eat ONE slice and FOUR chips. Then you eat TWO diet cookies. Now, don't reach for more. Don't eat for about four more hours. Then have a small snack of a small orange or apple with two Graham Crackers, and a glass of iced tea. If you eat like this for a while, you won't feel like you are even on a diet. You won't be hungry all of the time.

I chew sugarless gum. That really helps and the skim milk is good. You just get use to it. You eat half of everything. Drink tea, water, coffee, orange juice, skim milk, Graham Crackers, diet cookies – but only a few, wheat crackers, and watch the cheese. It's high in everything. Make up your own exercise program. Do the exercises about twice a day at first. Then do it once a week about the same time. You will feel different about four months down the road. You won't feel like you are on a diet. Get busy doing something or make crafts.

Don't spend all of your time in the kitchen. It's too close to the food. Go into the living room. You can't eat the couch. But if you did, then your guests would not have anything on which to sit. Get a grip on yourself and check out the menus.

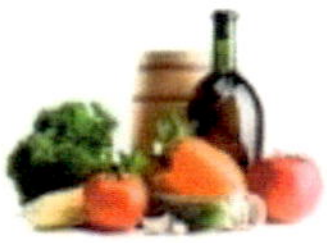

# Dandy Dieter

## *Recipes*

Eating healthy and doing exercises will be half of the battle. All you have to do is get off of the couch. Put your potato chips bag down. Walk past your glass of soda, and get in gear. Try this for a month, and stay close to the bathroom.

1. Medium leaf of lettuce
   1 tablespoon of tuna
   With onion
   1 teaspoon of Mayo
   Small tomato, sliced
   ½ slice of wheat bread
   6 grapes in 1 cup of yogurt
   ½ cup of sliced peaches
   8 oz. glass of iced tea

2. 1 egg with a slice of wheat bread
   Strawberry Jell-O with 6 grapes
   ½ cup of oatmeal
   Skim milk
   ½ cup of coffee

3. 2 Graham Crackers
   4 oz. glass of skimmed milk
   1 medium orange

Eat your heart out instead of making your hips go out.

4. ½ slice cucumber with a small tomato
   1 tablespoon of ranch dressing
   6 wheat crackers
   2 slices of baked turkey
   1 slice of wheat bread
   ½ cup of coffee

5. Small salad with tomato, onion, 1 cup of cucumber
   2 cups of onion soup
   3 slices of baked chicken (4 oz.)
   1 medium sliced apple
   8 oz. glass of iced water with lemon

6. 4 oz. baked fish with lemon
   1 cup of green beans
   1 small sweet potato
   1 teaspoon of butter
   1 cup of pineapple slices in orange Jell-O
   8 oz. of iced tea with lemon

Eat your heart out, instead of making your hips go out.

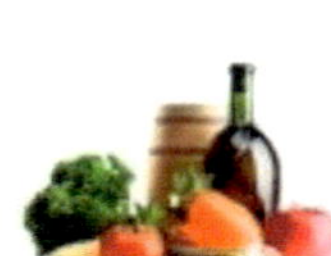

# Dandy Dieter

## *Recipes*

Well, how did you do with the first menus? Are you getting the idea yet? I put them together myself. I have been eating this way for three months now. I don't feel as if I'm on a diet, so the diet devil don't bother me. I have some more menus from which you may choose. Make up your own with the foods that you like. Merry, Merry Christmas here we come.

1. 1 slice of pizza
   1 cup of applesauce
   1 slice of watermelon (medium)
   ½ cup of strawberry yogurt
   2 diet cookies, sugar-free
   8 oz. glass of iced tea with lemon

2. 4 oz. hamburger on a bun
   ½ cup of slaw
   ½ cup of carrots
   1 medium banana
   4 oz. skimmed milk

3. ½ of a grilled cheese sandwich
   1 cup of tomato soup
   2 whole Graham Crackers with peanut butter spread
   4 wheat crackers
   Small orange
   Iced water or coffee

4. (Snack) 1 cup of strawberry Jell-O
   ½ cup of yogurt
   7 blackberries, no sugar
   4 grapes
   1 whole Graham Cracker section (4 squares)

5. (Snack) cut a cucumber
   Cut a tomato
   Cut some green peppers
   Chop an onion
   No salt, may use 1 tablespoon of Ranch Dressing

6. 1 medium sliced apple
   Cinnamon
   Heat in microwave

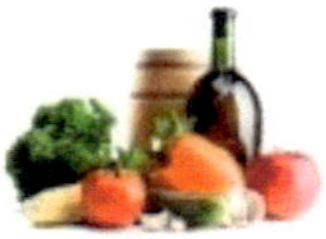

# Dandy Dieter

## *Recipes*

More menus are available for the thinner you. Pick the one that you like the most, and share it with others. How are you doing with the no-sweets and the no-cookies "by the bag" full?

Pretty soon you will be able to tighten your seat belt tighter. When your clothes start to hang on you, don't think something is wrong with you. It's just your thinner body finding its way out. I still say the best part of the day is when you can take your bra off. How about you gals?

If you are looking for something different to eat check these out.

1. 1 egg
   1 slice of wheat toast
   1 teaspoon of sugar-free jam
   2 slices of turkey bacon
   ½ cup of grapes
   Coffee

2. 1 cup of oatmeal
   1 slice of wheat toast
   Sugar-free jam
   1 small apple
   1 cup of coffee or skimmed milk

3. (Snack) 2 peanut butter crackers
   ½ slice of cucumber
   1 cup of iced water with lemon

4. 1 small baked chicken breast
   ½ cup of brown rice
   ½ cup of green beans
   1 slice of wheat bread
   1 cup of sliced pineapple
   8 oz. glass of iced tea

5. 1 medium cubed steak with sprinkled parsley
   ½ cup of steamed broccoli
   Small boiled potato with 1 teaspoon butter
   1 small sliced tomato
   ½ cup of blackberries

6. (Snack) 1 small peach
   1 cup of blueberry yogurt
   2 Graham Crackers

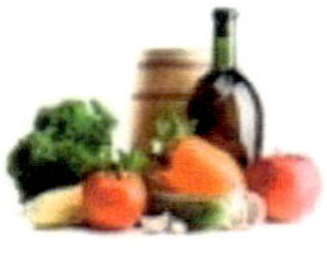

Chapter 17

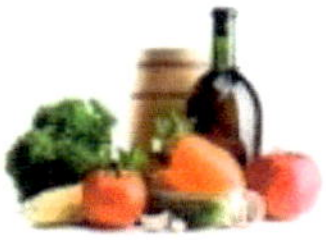

# Up The Ladder To Success

Are we still on the diet and trying this time?

You can't be a success by sitting on your buns. Giving up chips and donuts can be a real bummer, and don't forget to throw the brownies in the ditch. If you can't part with the brownies, and the donuts, you are in big trouble.

Let's talk about what will happen when you give up and eat as if you were a starving pit bull. You eat high calorie foods. You eat all the cookies that you want with whole milk because you don't like the taste of skim milk and never think about the fat or your blood sugar.

What a way to go "happy thighs". Next year at this time, you will be waddling from one room to the other. The brownies will be riding on your back side. How do you expect to get up the ladder by eating your face off? When you look in the mirror, you will look like a hamster, and your hair will look like your graduation picture.

Go on. Keep chewing on that ham and cheese sandwich. See if you don't wear a larger size for the holiday. We both know that you won't be going up the ladder, because you broke the first step with a hot dog hanging out of your mouth while trying to take a step.

God is watching you when you sneak the food into your bedroom at night. You will be bigger by morning. So eat a big breakfast. Is there anything that I can do to help you? I can always lock you in the closet until Christmas Eve. But I think that the family will miss you. There is hope even for you "Wide Pam". So get your mouth back on the diet and watch what you put in it. The ladder is not going to wait for you to make up your mind. Success is waiting for you.

Everybody that's on a diet knows that you have to try to get to another step. If you eat like a truck driver, it's just a ladder. A fat foot cannot step up for the ladder's step will break. You can diet with a friend, and see how much weight you can lose. Or you can give up and spend the holiday with the doctor because your body will be dragging.

Let me tell you about Dave and his two brothers, Jim and Joe. They were professional carpet installers and made an occupation out of it. Do you think that they became successful overnight? You know better. It took lots of hard work and many years.

They worked together. They taught each other. They did private and commercial work. They had setbacks and the business was slow at times. But did they give up? No. They kept going and don't you think that their knees and their backs hurt? You bet they did. How do you think they got to the top of the ladder? They worked hard to be successful and it paid off.

Let's take the dieter who can't get on the first step of the ladder. We have Karen who can't get her heavy foot on the ladder. She has been on so many diets just as many peas in one can. Karen is not active, eats anything she wants, and walks really slowly. She is over-weight.

Do you think that Karen is going up the ladder of success? I don't think so. How can we help Karen to be a success, and lose some weight? Do we pull her off of the couch with a rope? Do we knock the fast food out of her hands? Or do we just pray and ask God to push her half way up the ladder?

There are miracles, but there is not one where your fat just falls on the floor all by itself. If there is, how much does it cost? Every dieter in the world would like one of those miracles, I'm sure.

So we know that the three brothers didn't become successful overnight. Hard work comes with a pay-off. Dieters' payoff is when they reach their goal. There are a lot of successful people on the top of the ladder. I wonder how many dieters are up there. You could be one of them.

Do it for yourself. Don't do a lose-weight-fast diet. You will just gain it all back. On your way up the ladder, take a brush with you. When you get up to the top, paint the ceiling while you are up there. The ladder of success is for anybody. Some make it, and some never get to the first step. I'm sure that at times those brothers felt like giving up, but I bet they are glad they didn't.

How many dieters out there are going to give it their best shot? I wonder, will one of them be you? All I have to say is "Get up on that ladder and climb. By the time you get back down on the ground, you will be thinner, Praise God."

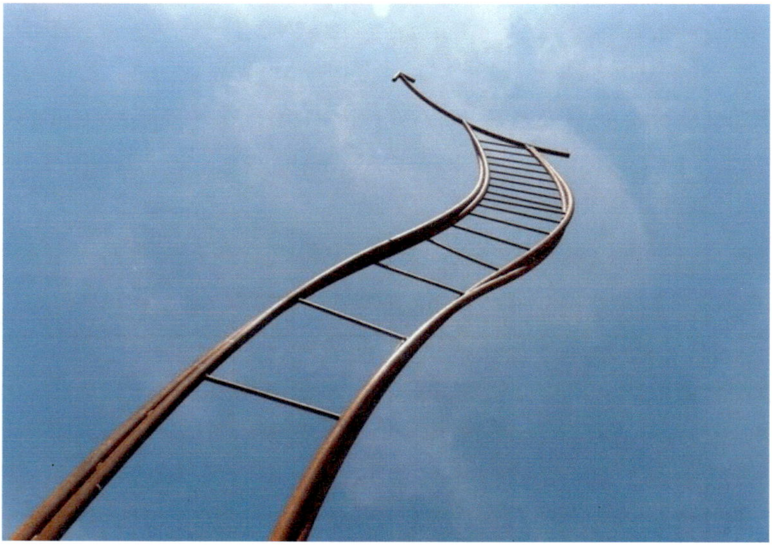

Jacob's ladder (Pixabay.com)

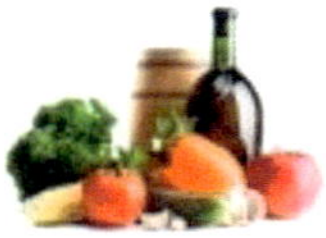

Chapter 18

# Reasons Why You Can't Lose Weight

The doctor has heard all of the excuses why you can't lose any weight. Some of them are pretty funny. How about the one that "All of the people in my family are heavy and have a problem losing weight."

I like the one who said, "Doctor, will you check my hormones?"

What about the one, "I have tried so hard and only lost three pounds."

How about this one? "I think that my scale is broken."

I have to share this one with you. I do feel like a fool. I was really trying to go on a diet. I went to weigh myself and I thought "Woo baby, this can't be true." I went to work the next day and couldn't get that off my mind. I was talking to a co-worker when no one was around us.

I said to her, "You know, I lost twenty pounds." I noticed the look that she gave me, but she just said, "That's real good." I felt pretty good for the rest of the day. I then went back and got the scale and got back on it. To my surprise, the darn scale was really broken. Boy, did we laugh. It made our whole day. I know that if she reads my book, she will remember that one story for sure.

Life will get better. We just have to keep patience until then. You can't worry about what you can't change. Just work on what you can change. In time, things will work out.

What is your reason why you can't lose weight? Do you think this is easy? Not by a far shot. Rain is like losing weight. You never know how much weight you will gain, and how long it will be before it stops.

Lose weight when you are young. When you get older, you will need God on your side for help. You can always say that you can't lose weight because, when you exercise, you always hurt your back. Did you ever say that one? I'm sure you have a reason that you've been using for years. Lose some weight so you won't have to say it next year. That will be a happy year.

How do you know that you are being honest with yourself? You have had so many excuses for why your diet didn't work. Maybe God made you with different clay, and gave you a little extra. You do know that you have to really try, don't you? Fat is not going to go away like a bad dream.

When you sit on the couch, and one side goes up in the air, that's a good sign that you need to be on a diet. You have to learn how to control yourself when you are alone. Don't think that you can eat like a starving puppy. I can't wait for about three months to hear your excuse for eating the donut in your mouth, and why your diet was so bad.

I wonder if you will use the same one that you used on the last diet, or make up another one. You have to think thin to be thin. Try looking at a really heavy person. You can't picture yourself in that shape. Maybe you are only a few pounds higher, or lower than that person. Now what do you think?

I like the excuse that my neighbor gave me last summer when she tried a new diet. I think that she was on the diet for about six months. I then noticed that she was losing a little weight and looking nice.

A few days later, I saw her carrying in groceries and it looked as if she was feeding a small army. I then asked her about her diet. You better sit down on this one. She said that the diet was no good for her. It kept giving her too much gas, and she was stinking up the kitchen. Please pass the box of tissue. I think this one was the very best.

If you can beat that one, let's hear it. You can tell your favorite excuse to make yourself feel better, but do you think anybody is going to buy it? When you lose the weight, people will notice it and tell you. Now that will make you feel good.

So have you bought your new outfit for Christmas yet? This will be a holiday to remember. I knew that you could do it. I just had to gripe at you enough to get you going. This book is going to help you to focus on yourself. You have helped so many others. Now is the time to do something for yourself. You are worth it, and you deserve to be proud of yourself. Life is too short to eat like a bird for the rest of your life. Now after reading this book, you know that you don't have to do so. Thank you Jesus!

Well, here we go again, trying to get rid of the backside without hurting ourselves. Have you thought of another reason why you can't seem to lose weight? I heard some pretty good ones, and I know that you are sick of this whole diet thing. Well count me in.

I lost fifteen (15) pounds in two months. I will not give up until my jeans fall past my knees. I want this Christmas to be one to remember. So how are you doing with the fast food that you can't eat? To be honest with you, I sure miss the hamburgers and fries. The chocolate is driving me nuts.

I knew a girl who lost ten pounds and then would reward herself by eating two ice creams. Yet she couldn't figure out why it took her a whole year to lose twenty pounds.

You don't need an excuse when you eat anything you want. Can you think of an excuse someone gave you for not losing weight? Was it the same one you used for not losing? Just pass them around. Maybe you can sell your excuses to all of the dieters, and start up a little business. We have heard everything including "I just get so tired of diets and exercises".

I guess some people would rather eat the good stuff than look nice and be thin. We don't get everything we want in life. That's what makes life a challenge.

Do you know anybody who is heavier than you? Would you like to see them in the grocery store and see them a lot smaller than you? I'm sure you would think, how did they do that – not overnight, I'm sure?

Can you think of how proud that person is of herself? So as far as the heavy weights go, with God's help, we will be thin. So back off, you skinny people. Here we come.

Is there anything you would like to say to the skinny people? Here is your chance. Remember, by eating less bread, you will get thinner and at the end, you will be a winner. Say your little fat prayer, now and then.

"Please Lord, may only healthy foods go through my lips, and all of the good food go into the ditch."

Say this prayer every night before bedtime. In time, with hard work, you will lose weight. Let others use all of the excuses, and go to bed with a donut under their pillow. Now if you go to bed with a donut under your pillow, there is no hope for you, and when you wake up, it will be harder to get out of bed. Enjoy your donut.

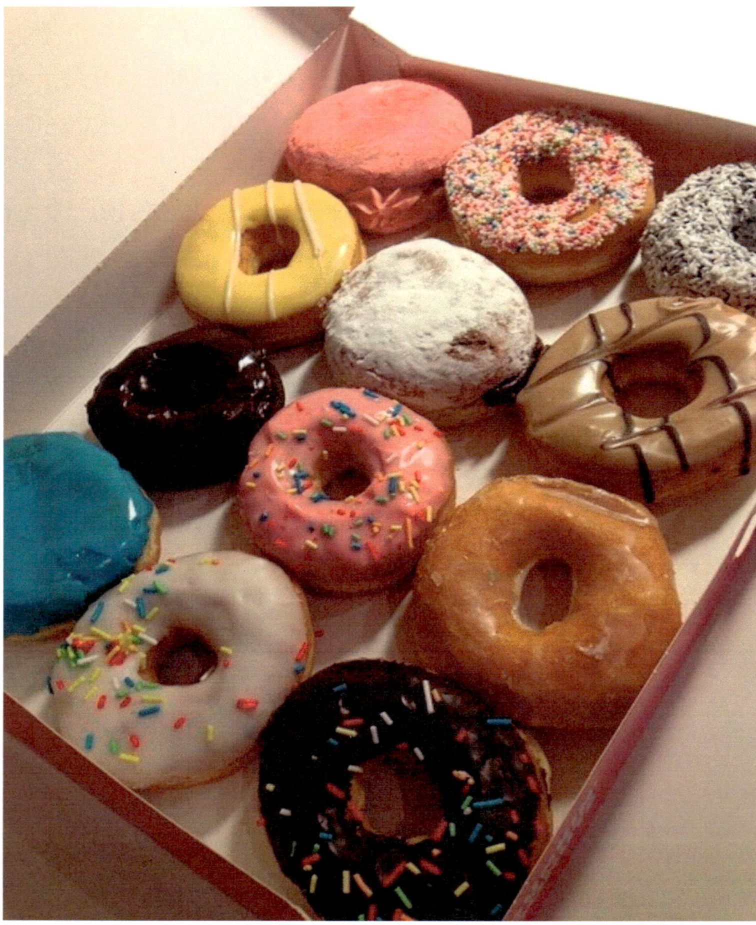

One Reason Why You Can't Lose Weight

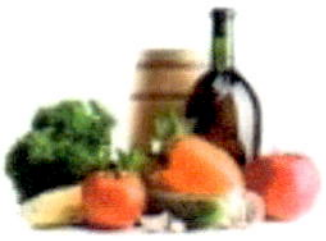

Chapter 19

# Ribbons for Losers

Did you know that you could be a winner and a loser at the same time? Think about that for a moment. If you work hard and lose weight, you get a ribbon for losing and when you get a ribbon, you are a winner. My question is, "How many ribbons do you want? How about all of them?" You will get a red ribbon when you lose ten pounds, and a green one for fifteen pounds. At least you will feel that you are losing weight for a purpose – for a ribbon and a thinner body.

If you happen to lose twenty-eight or more pounds you will get a pink ribbon. By that time you should be in the pink. When you reach your goal, you will get a gold ribbon.

I have a green ribbon, and three pounds from getting a pink one. Let me tell you, some days I would rather have a slice of pizza than a ribbon. You can't eat the ribbon. Well maybe some do – those who are having trouble with their sweets.

How are we doing so far? Are you ready for a beer? It sounds good but you better drink water to be on the safe side.

I saw Ann Miller at the store the other day. I met Ann at a New Year's Eve party about eight years ago. Ann is married to David. Ann has been trying to lose weight for as long as I have known her. I think she found a good diet for her this time. She told me that she had lost thirty pounds, and boy did it look nice with her blonde hair.

She had worked very hard to look that nice. That could be you. We talked for a while and then she had to get going. It was nice to see the happy look on her face. You see, hard work does pay off if you really try.

How are you doing with the cookies? They could make you lose your mind if you let them. You can always freeze all of the candy and give it out next trick or treat day. Don't forget to thaw it out. I just loved trick or treat. I could make a Milkyway disappear faster than you could blink an eye. It's not as fun trying to make a carrot disappear, but your body will reward you with a thinner behind.

I was at the post office and saw Sara and her husband John. I have known Sara for about twenty years and I went to her wedding when she married John. Sara told me that she had lost forty-seven pounds. She looked so nice and she looked like a different person. John just smiled when he looked at her. It took her ten months to lose the weight, and she did it very well.

That goes to show you that when you try, sometimes the whole world is trying to lose weight. I know that at times you have lost maybe fifty pounds and then gained back more weight. Well climb in the boat with the rest of us.

Being healthy is one thing, but eating healthy is a whole new ball game. Do I have any hands in the air? I thought so. Is anybody doing their exercise daily? I better get going on that one. When I raise my arm up, my flab waves before my hand does. When I walk too fast, my legs feel like they are flapping in the wind. My fat must be loose.

Things happen when you lose weight. You notice your arms seem to be hanging when they didn't before. When you sit on a chair, it feels as if you are on a bone. Your fat is slowly moving around. You have to exercise to keep the fat in the right place. Or when you drive down the highway, and some kid yells "Hey grandma, get off the road!" You look around and realize that they are yelling at you.

Exercise class starts in ten minutes. Be there. This book is not to put anybody down. It's just that it seems like everybody is having trouble trying to trim down. Let's face it, there is nothing funny about trying to lose weight.

You hear about people who have lost a hundred pounds, and you wonder how they did that. You know that it took many long months to lose that much weight. Somebody told me that the more you sweat, the more weight that you lose. What do you think about that one?

Carrots are good for you but they are not the answer. You have to eat the right vegetables with them. Mine is Spinach. I just love Spinach and cabbage. They are the best. Do you know some good recipes that you could share with others? Why don't we trade off recipes and give dieters a variety from which to choose. Then we can help each other, and make friends along the way. There are over a hundred books on diets. Nobody likes to read about being heavy. They know it, but they will read about how others lost weight to give them ideas that might help them.

Do you feel as if you are eating the same food all of the time? That would get pretty boring. I would like to share some of the recipes that my friends gave me that you might like to try.

The one that I eat a lot is Cabbage Soup.

1. Boil a small head of cabbage.
2. Drain a can of green beans, corn, carrots, and put them into the pan with the cabbage.
3. Slice a can of whole potatoes. Rinse with cold water and then add to the cabbage mixture.
4. I add a can of stewed tomatoes, but it's to be used if you like tomatoes.
5. At the same time that you cook the cabbage mixture, use another pan and

cook ½ pound of stew meat with chopped celery until tender.

6. Drain the stew meat and add to the cabbage.
7. Stir the mixture.
8. Get a bowl. Put in the soup and eat with four wheat crackers and a glass of skim milk. Enjoy.

You will like this because it is full of vitamins, and it fills you up. What are you having for dinner? Try the next one for lunch.

Rinse a whole leaf of lettuce. Fix one can of tuna with chopped onion, and one teaspoon of mayonnaise. Put the lettuce on a plate, with two tablespoons of tuna in it. Put in a small sliced tomato. Eat with four wheat crackers and one-half cup of applesauce, with a small sliced apple. Are you getting hungry yet?

Breakfast is the most important meal of the day. We should have a full one to start the day. Remember to eat small portions and save the extra calories. Try this for breakfast, and see what you think.

1. One boiled egg with one slice of wheat toast
2. A small sliced tomato
3. Two slices of turkey bacon
4. A small orange and a cup of coffee with light cream

You can eat a snack about four and one-half hours later. Fix this for the snack:

1. One cup of strawberry yogurt
2. One cup of strawberry Jell-O with a few strawberries
3. One Graham Cracker

This one I really like. You only have to eat it once and you will see how good it is. Now for the snack that you can pick in between meals.

1. Get a medium container with a lid.
2. Pop one fat-free popcorn
3. Get one cup of raisins brand cereal
4. I add up to five Graham Crackers with a cup of unsalted pretzels.

This is just a snack, not a meal. So don't eat until it's empty. Save some for later.

Some things that you can eat to break your hunger are apples, a peach, three carrots with a very little ranch dressing, one cup of sliced cucumbers, a slice of fat-free cheese with two wheat crackers. I hope that I gave you a few new ideas to help you along the way. Good luck, and enjoy the cabbage.

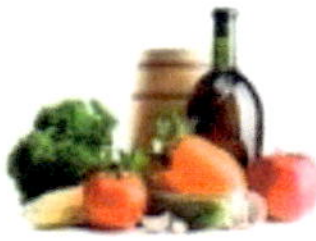

Chapter 20

# Surprise Yourself And Lose Weight

I hope that I have encouraged a few people to get serious about losing some weight.

I am not going to tell you that this is easy. We are all on the same fishing trip, fishing for the right answers. We are floating in the same boat. By the way, I don't even like to fish.

I don't know all of the answers. I'm just trying to turn some couch potatoes into hot potatoes. I'm not talking about hot flashes.

You always heard that you are what you eat. Well, who wants to be built like a double burger with cheese? Do you know the real value of a carrot and a slice of cucumber? It will fill you up and it sure is good for you.

Have you gotten into an outfit that your hips haven't gotten into for the past five years? That should tell you that you are doing something right.

Do you still have a smile on your face? Notice that when you gain a few pounds, people look at you and then turn away? They are surprised and don't want to say anything to hurt your feelings.

Think of the look on their face when you lose about forty pounds, and walk through the door.

You get to see their faces and feel proud of yourself.

How are you doing with your diet? Did you see any good snacks in this book? Are you sharing any tips that will help others? This is the best way to diet and you won't feel as if the whole world is against you.

Think of how you will feel when you reach your goal. You can make up new dishes and eat half of what you normally eat. Watch the sugar and the calories. You won't even miss the old way you use to eat. After a while, you will be half of the body that you use to be.

Everybody in the world wants to be thin. Why not you?

This is your year for a nice miracle and the reward of smaller outfits. I think that you will do just fine. You will surprise yourself and everybody around you when you strut your stuff.

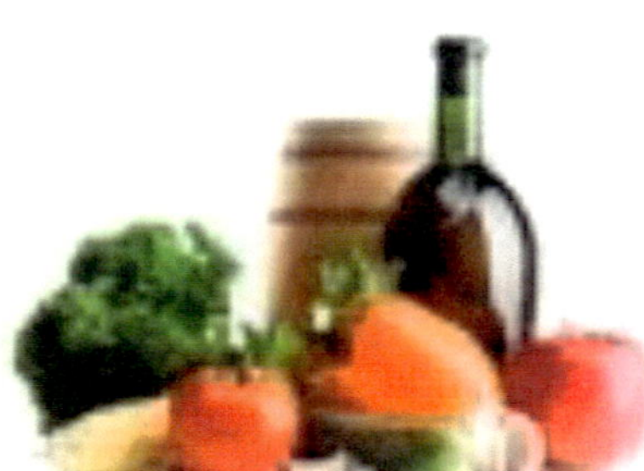

Have Carrots, Will Travel, And Grab Yourself An Apple.

# Author's View

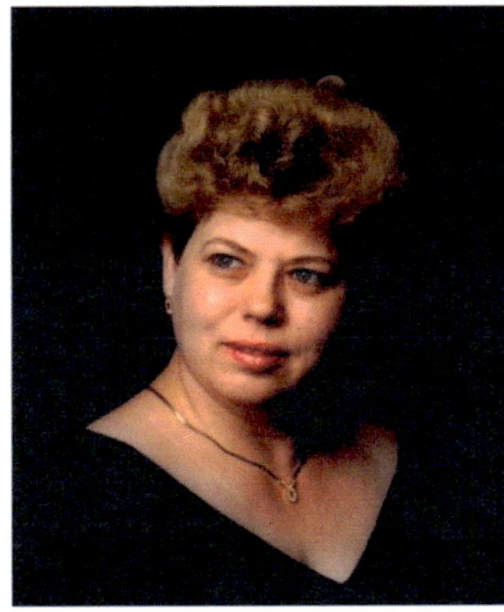

Hello. My name is Judy Schwartz. I am a published author and a songwriter. I was born and reared in Saint Louis, Missouri.

I graduated from Riverview Gardens Senior High School. I always enjoyed reading poetry and verses.
I wrote an inspirational book of poetry entitled Special Thoughts For Special People. I created my own book cover and designed the art on each page.

You can view my book at the e-store -
https://www.createspace.com/3378210.
I have always been grateful for my freedom and I do thank our soldiers.
When I thought of all the parents that lost a child in the awful war, I gained an idea. I decided to write two songs for soldiers. I felt the need to honor our heroes, and to give the parents closure.

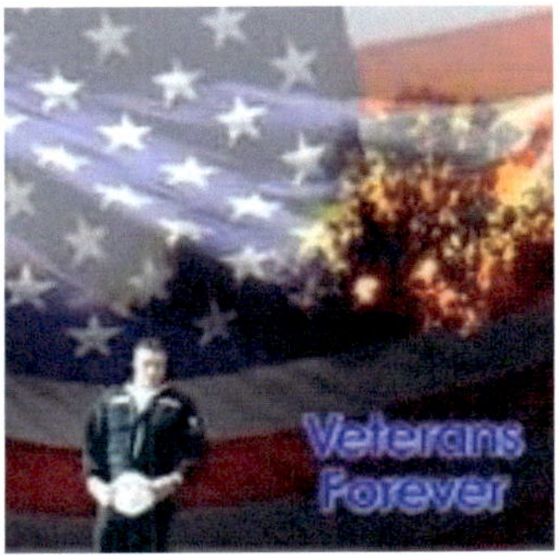


The first song is entitled "The Proud Hero".
When I wrote the lyrics, I covered land, air and sea. Therefore, the second song is called "Heavenly Love".
(left) James Jacobs, sailor A S 3 James D Jacobs U. S. A.

The soldier's voice in the song is singing from Heaven. This song will touch your heart.

Arthur McClendon is the music composer and singer who is playing a grand piano in the video. When you view the video, it will mesmerize you.

If you have any questions about getting a CD, please e-mail me jude20@sbcglobal.net.

Special Thoughts For Special People*
by
Judy Schwartz (Judith Ann Schwartz)

My book of inspirational readings will touch your heart and make a fine gift for that special someone. Don't forget that you may find it at http://www.createspace.com/3378210. The book is a keepsake item. You will need to read it over and over once you select your favorite page. Thanks again.
Judy

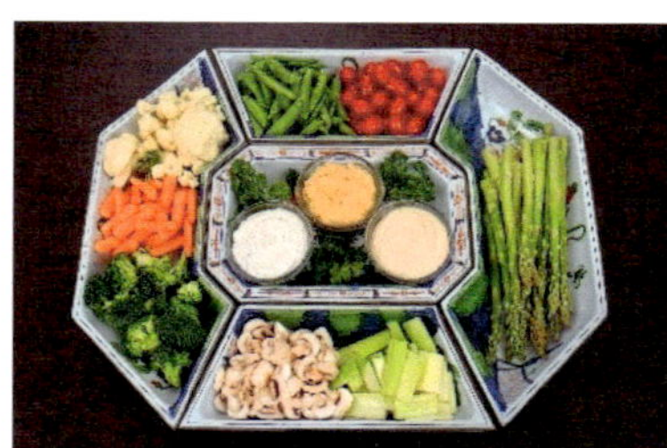

Made in the USA
Las Vegas, NV
10 November 2026

57845501R00071